MUZZLED TRUTH

How the California Department of Public Health Rejected COVID-19 Treatment and Vaccine Health Risks Warnings

MUZZLED TRUTH

How the California Department of Public Health Rejected COVID-19 Treatment and Vaccine Health Risks Warnings

Ronald F. Owens Jr.

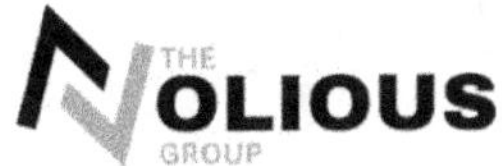

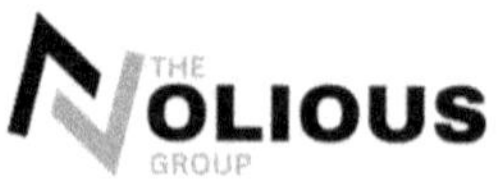

Dedicated to Dr. Barbara E. Cahoon-Young,

mother of Stephanie E. Owens and mother-in-law

of my brother Leonard E. Owens.

Dr. Cahoon-Young, who retired as Placer County Public Health Lab Director on July 14, 2010, may have died from COVID-19 vaccines on July 4, 2021.

"Document, document, document!"
—Ronald F. Owens Sr.

*"Withhold not good from them to whom it is due,
when it is in the power of thine hand to do it."*

—Proverbs 3:27

FOREWORD

When the first reports emerged from Wuhan, China, of a virulent, highly infectious respiratory disease afflicting thousands of people, I was alarmed. Having worked for many years in California's State Department of Public Health (CDPH) in the aftermath of the 9/11 attacks, I paid close attention to any news reports of unusual disease activity. The more I heard the reports from Wuhan, the more I was convinced that this was a serious outbreak and a real threat to public health.

By that time, I was retired from my position as the Department's Assistant Chief Counsel for Contracts and Prevention Services. I was no longer supervising the lawyers who advised the public health programs or preparing training materials on the law pertaining to emergency preparedness or communicable disease control. I fully expected to see my former employer and the federal Centers for Disease Control exercise their authority to prevent or, at least, slow the introduction of this apparently new pathogen into the United States and California.

And so it was with increasing alarm that I watched as little or nothing of the sort occurred. The airports continued to receive flights from China, and even after flights from Wuhan were stopped, they continued to arrive from other cities in China and other Asian countries, often carrying potentially infected people from the Wuhan region. It was as if public health officials were waiting until the disease, reportedly highly infectious and spread by droplet or aerosol transmission, was established within the US before taking action.

When public health finally did act, it was to impose lockdowns for two weeks to slow the spread and prevent hospitals from being overwhelmed, they said. This kind of civil detention of people in the absence of any evidence that they were infected or had even been exposed was unprecedented and contrary to the law. "What in the world," I wondered, "was going on at CDPH?"

I retreated to the rural property I owned, watched, and waited. I had no television reception there and resorted to sources on the Internet to track the outbreak's progress and gather information on the disease itself.

At this point, I was fully persuaded that the disease was real, potentially lethal, particularly to the elderly like myself, spread via aerosol transmission, and was spreading rapidly. I believed that masks might be effective over the short run in reducing the severity of disease cases by reducing the potential viral inoculation dose and even spent many late winter hours at a sewing machine making masks for myself and friends.

It first dawned on me that things might not be at all what they seemed when I observed the media and the "scientific" response to President Donald Trump's messaging about chloroquine and hydroxychloroquine as potential treatments of this new disease, now denominated as "COVID-19." These were inexpensive, off-patent, widely available drugs with a long track record of human use without significant adverse effects. Dr. Anthony Fauci had himself proclaimed these to be miracle drugs in treating earlier coronavirus outbreaks. "What harm could there be," I thought, "in giving these treatments a try?"

But rather than be encouraged, grateful, or even curious whether these drugs might be effective against COVID-19, President Trump's detractors and the media attacked him in unison for even suggesting it. Even the drugs themselves were attacked. So-called "scientists" went so far as to conjure up fraudulent studies to disprove the effectiveness of these drugs. The media cited these studies long after they had been shown to be entirely fraudulent. [1] [2] [3] I began to wonder if these people had any genuine interest in saving lives.

I watched this process repeated when ivermectin emerged as an even more effective treatment. This inexpensive, widely-available drug used to treat both humans and animals for various conditions proved to be highly effective in treating COVID-19 infections, even in severe cases. Once again, the media attacked the drug, disparaged as a "horse dewormer," and blocked from use as a COVID-19 treatment by various governmental agencies. This included CDPH, which went to great lengths to discourage the public from using veterinary formulations of ivermectin while turning a blind eye to the fact that other

---

[1] Sarah Boseley and Melisa Davey, "Covid-19: Lancet retracts paper that halted hydroxychloroquine trials," The Guardian, June 4, 2020.

[2] Mandeep R Mehra, Frank Ruschitzka, Amit N Patel, "Retraction—Hydroxychloroquine or chloroquine with or without a macrolide for treatment of COVID-19: a multinational registry analysis," The Lancet, June 5, 2020.

[3] Patrice Wendling, "Despite Retraction, Study Using Fraudulent Surgisphere Data Still Cited," Medscape Medical News, August 5, 2021.

state agencies were preventing public and medical professional access to formulations of the drug appropriate for humans.

By now, it was obvious that neither the media, the public health agencies, nor the medical/industrial establishment had any interest in finding or utilizing effective legacy drugs or saving lives. At the beginning of 2021, it became apparent why. Vaccines had been developed and would be dispensed under "emergency use authorizations" from the Food and Drug Administration, something that can only occur in the absence of effective treatments of the target infection. And there was a lot of money to be made.

I had serious doubts that a safe and effective vaccine could have been developed in such a short period of time and recalled from the SARS-COV1 outbreak of 2003 that making such a vaccine against coronaviruses had not previously been successful. I immediately decided to not vaccinate and wait, and I encouraged my family and friends to do the same. Few listened.

I watched as nurse Tiffany Dover collapsed after receiving her injection. I watched as videos emerged showing people suffering from uncontrollable whole-body tremors that went on for days or weeks after vaccination. I watched in horror as the number of adverse events, including deaths, reported to the Centers for Disease Control and Prevention (CDC) through its Vaccine Adverse Event Reporting System (VAERS) soared into the thousands.

And while visiting Sacramento in August 2021, I heard a public service announcement (PSA), brought to you by CDPH, stating that the COVID-19 vaccines had been proven to be safe and effective. I knew this to be a complete and utter lie.

I sent a Public Records Act (PRA) request to CDPH seeking records pertaining to this PSA. I wanted to know who within CDPH had authorized or approved such a claim. What I learned through the response was that no one in CDPH had done so. CDPH had simply given $40 million dollars to a San Francisco advertising agency, which had created the PSA without any apparent review by CDPH, and put it on air.

By some strange twist of fate, my PRA request was erroneously forwarded to Ron Owens, with whom I had been acquainted prior to my retirement and who still worked in the CDPH Office of Communications. We reconnected over our mutual concern that public health officials were failing to protect, and even harming, public health.

Of course, from my rural, isolated perch in retirement, I was never subjected to the pressures of those still working at CDPH who had come to the same realization. I never had to worry that raising my concerns might jeopardize my employment. I never had to endure a staff meeting in which managers embraced the increasingly obvious lies and spin of the mainstream media or congratulated themselves on a job well done in the face of growing evidence that flawed policies were harming members of the public. I never had to listen to group-thinking bureaucrats brand "conspiracy theories" or dismiss as untrustworthy the reports of vaccine injuries and deaths now thoroughly documented in VAERS. I never had to personally witness those who had taken an oath to support and defend and to bear true faith and allegiance to both the United States and California Constitutions violate those oaths by conspiring to silence or censor any view contrary to their own, calling it misinformation or disinformation, in direct violation of the right to freedom of speech.

I have often wondered whether, had my circumstances been different, I would have had the same courage that Mr. Owens displayed. Would I have spoken out in my dismay and rising anger over what was obviously becoming a public health catastrophe? Would I have risked being "canceled" to inject what I perceived to be the awful truth into CDPH's self-approving narrative? I will, of course, never know, but I like to think that, like Mr. Owens, I would have spoken out and acted on behalf of the public that the public health profession ostensibly serves.

I often reflect on former colleagues still working for CDPH in leadership positions who apparently lacked that same courage. Did they truly believe what could easily be seen to be completely false? Did they willingly enforce policies that were, in fact, harmful to the public? Were they somehow compromised through threats or bribery? Or were they simply too afraid or submissive to attempt to alter the trajectory set by those in power, thinking it was better to stay silent and remain employed even if doing harm, choosing personal prosperity over public responsibility?

I believe that the day will come when public health officials and professionals will be held to account for their acts and omissions during the so-called COVID-19 pandemic. What transpired was nothing short of murder on a colossal scale in which they played a substantial role.

Millions were victimized, initially by a pathogen intentionally developed in a laboratory under the guise of public health protection and subsequently by the public health response. Millions were subjected to fear created by false statistics based on inappropriate PCR tests promoted by public health officials. The infected were denied early and effective treatments like ivermectin, again by public health officials. They were subjected to ineffective and even deadly treatment protocols administered by hospitals under public health supervision. They were injured or killed by an untested and unsafe "vaccine" actively promoted by public health officials. Many undoubtedly succumbed to bacterial infections acquired by complying with mask mandates. And millions were made victims of poverty, despair, and isolation inflicted by illegal public health measures, particularly the lockdowns. To be sure, many others were involved, but public health played a central role in this murderous campaign.

When that justice comes, I hope Mr. Owens and I are alive to see it.

—Peter A. Baldridge
October 7, 2023

(Peter A. Baldridge served as the Assistant Chief Counsel for the California Department of Public Health from 2009-2014. From 1987 to 2009 Mr. Baldridge advised public and environmental health agencies of the State as an attorney, and served as the Chief Counsel of the Office of Environmental Health Hazard Assessment from 1991 to 1993. He began his state service in the Office of the State Controller from 1982 to 1987. He is a graduate of the University of the South, Sewanee, Tennessee and the University of the Pacific McGeorge School of Law, Sacramento, California. He is retired and currently practices fire-risk reduction on 15 acres in the Sierra foothills.)

CONTENTS

PREFACE

It was she, Dora L. Owens, who delivered her seven-pound, six-ounce and twenty-inch-long baby at the Air Force Hospital at Tachikawa, Japan. Her husband, SSgt. Ronald F. Owens, was a French horn player assigned to the Air Force Band at Yomato Air Station. Their second child was taken to the nursery. She rested comfortably in her bed, but a nurse brought their newborn son back to the twenty-five-year-old mother. Puzzled, the mother asked why the nurse returned her newborn son. The nurse said the baby kept crying. The nurse also said the baby's crying awoke other babies in the nursery. Who knows how long Dora's and Ronald's firstborn son kept the other babies awake?

Yes, you guessed correctly; that newborn baby was me.

Many times, my late eighty-nine-year-old mother shared about me crying and waking other babies in the nursery. Ever since her June 13, 2021, passing—she died at home in bed clasping my dad's right hand and holding my left hand—I have often thought about this story.

That incident that happened more than sixty-six years ago when I was a baby illustrates what I attempted to do the past couple years as an adult. Just as I literally cried and awoke babies at Tachikawa's hospital in 1957, I figuratively cried and tried to awake babies at the California Department of Public Health between 2021 and 2023.

INTRODUCTION

Figuratively crying to awake the babies at the California Department of Public Health (CDPH) was foremost on my mind on August 26, 2023. That Saturday, I walked 4.4 miles at a park. This twenty-one-acre park is near where I currently live, and a nice 0.5-mile pedestrian track encircles part of it.

Between 10 a.m. and noon that day, I slowly walked more than eight laps around that hardpan track. I held my iPhone in my right hand, spoke into the microphone, and recorded one hour and twenty-eight minutes of monologue in a transcription app. It was a physically energetic exercise period and an emotionally cathartic recording session. During that recording, I reported what I thought, felt, observed, and experienced as a CDPH Information Officer 2. That recording laid the foundation of this book.

I had been employed at CDPH's Office of Public Affairs—now Office of Communications—since March 2, 2009.

Yes, a couple CDPH Deputy Directors wrote me up for not meeting expectations. Yes, I was challenged proofreading daily media update reports. Yes, I didn't see a couple of Public Record Act (PRA) request emails that came in my basket. And yes, I got in trouble because I didn't respond to these PRA requestors by the mandated ten days of their dated emails.

But for the most part, I was a good, trusted, hard-working, honest, and, yes, a generous employee.

I donated more than five gallons of blood at the local blood bank throughout my state civil service career. I was a United Way California State Employees Charitable Campaign (now branded Our Promise) payroll deduction donor. I even lent my vocal and whistling talents in several annual CDPH food drive talent shows. For example, there's a YouTube video of me whistling the woodwind instrument of George Frideric Handel's La Rèjouissance from Music for the Royal Fireworks in 2012 before 250 CDPH employees.[4]

At the writing of this book, I am at the sunset of a nearly thirty-year state service career and less than six months away from commemorating my fifteen-year anniversary at CDPH. I am the most tenured, experienced, and, at more than sixty-six years old, probably the eldest Office of Communications staff member.

I believe that since much is given from God, my parents and myself (through good choices), my coworkers, my superiors, reporters, and most importantly 40 million Californians require much.

Thus, it was incumbent upon me, a seasoned CDPH employee who strived to do the right thing in life, to have revealed—in a series of emails—to my superiors between October 2021 to October 2023 these two revelations:

1. Properly dosed human ivermectin cures COVID-19.

---

[4] Ron Owens whistling the La Rèjouissance for Music | Royal Fireworks, by George Frideric Handel, last modified on April 12, 2013.

2. COVID-19 vaccines are "killing people . . ." and have not been "safe and effective" for millions of people.

I shared these two revelations with CDPH's powers that be, but I was unsuccessful in getting them to listen to me. Undeterred, I decided to share with the general public these two revelations plus a lot more in this book, which is based on my dad's "document, document, document" things that happen in the workplace sage advice.

This is not the first time I have written a book. If this had been my first book, that inexperience would have inhibited me, the writer and narrator, and had been detrimental to you, the Reader or Listener. Up to this point, I have written five books—while being the caregiver of my late 106-year-old maternal grandmother (Lovelei C. Sterling) and late 89-year-old mother (Dora L. Owens.)

In four books, I figuratively insert my feet in the sandals of Bible characters and tell their stories in their own words. In one book, I posit myself as an observer and report Bible stories.

In *Noah, Preparer of the Ark,* I strap my feet in the sandals of Noah. It was I, Noah, who will share how I built the ark and how my family survived the great global flood.

In *Judas, Betrayer of Jesus,* I slip my feet in Judas's sandals. It was I, Judas, who will share why I betrayed Jesus, how I betrayed Jesus, and the consequences of betraying Jesus.

In *Story of Rich Man and Lazarus: Hell and Heaven Described in Their Own Words,* I fit my pedicured, pampered feet in the alligator shoes of a billionaire and lace my boots in the crusted, unkempt feet of a homeless man. I share how they lived, died, and where they spent eternity. It was I, a certain rich man, who dressed well, ate well, lived well, and made lots of money. It was I, a certain homeless man who dressed poorly, ate uneaten food, lived on the city streets, and had very little money.

In "*Lucifer, Enemy of God*, I write an Old Testament overview and introduce my flagship book about people who were directly or indirectly involved with and impacted by Jesus the Christ.

In *Spectators of Jesus the Christ*, I insert my feet in the sandals of twenty-six people—seventeen men and nine women. I share their imagined thoughts, perceived feelings, and fictional observations of Jesus's life, teachings, miracles, and redemptive power. I was blessed that Evangelist Alveda C. King, a niece of Dr. Martin Luther King Jr., wrote the foreword of my flagship book. (Please note that my *Lucifer* book is chapter 1 of *Spectators*, and my *Judas* book are chapters 21, 23, and 24 of *Spectators*.)

My fictional first-person scriptural writings are based on *The Holy Bible*. All five of my books are published in paperback and eBook. Just as I narrated my four other books in the walk-in closet at home, I narrated this book at home as well. My books—excluding *Lucifer, Enemy of God*— are available on iTunes or Audible. These *Bible*-based books, which are on my <**www.RonaldFOwensJr.com**> website, represent "a new and innovative genre of Christian literature."[5]

My *Muzzled Truth: How the California Department of Public Health Rejected COVID-19 Treatment and Vaccine Health Risks Warnings* represents that same first-person literary storytelling technique. *Muzzled Truth* is based on my professional career and CDPH experience

---

[5] Google Ronald F. Owens Jr. website.

before, during and after the COVID-19 pandemic. In this book, I am literally inserting my feet in my own shoes and am telling my thoughts, feelings, observations, and experiences in my own words.

So just as I have written "It was I…" when identifying the names and introducing the characters in my other books, I do so here and now . . .

It was I, Luke, who was a bright-eyed and energetic big baby boy when I was born to my parents, but my body changed after doctors and nurses needled me…

And…

It was I, Ronald Owens, who emailed California Department of Public Health (CDPH) leadership and notified them a Biden Administration health official said that COVID-19 vaccines are killing people of color at about two times the rate of White Americans.

But CDPH's Office of Communications management initially ignored me, subsequently threatened disciplinary action against me, rudely muzzled me, and, finally, gaslighted me.

Dear Reader or Listener, thank you for reading or listening to *Muzzled Truth*. I purposely capitalized "Reader" or "Listener" out of respect for you, your name, your interest, and your time.

CHAPTER 1
Klingerman Foundation Lesson

It was I, a Department of Motor Vehicles Media Relations Office staffer, who learned to ascertain the veracity of information sent from a credible and trusted governmental official before believing it.

Midway through my tenure as a DMV Information Officer 1, I received an email from a former boss during the week of September 3, 2001. She supervised me for four years when I worked as one of the Department of Toxic Substances Control's Office of Military Facilities' Public Participation Specialist.

The email she sent warned recipients that if we received a blue envelope in the mail addressed from the Klingerman Foundation, we were not to open it. That Klingerman Foundation envelope was laced with a toxic white powder and had contaminated and killed twenty-three people.

Even though I had not heard of any mainstream media reports about twenty-three people being contaminated, sickened, and died by toxic white powder, I still deemed this Klingerman Foundation envelope email credible because of the source.

So I selected eleven DMV recipients. I forwarded them that Klingerman Foundation email. "Ron Owens, Public Information Officer, Department of Motor Vehicles, phone number and email address" was displayed in my signature block at the bottom of my email.

I also blind-copied my sister, a California Department of Corrections and Rehabilitation employee. Shortly thereafter, my sister called and said Snopes, an urban legends reference page, determined the Klingerman Foundation email was a hoax.

I thanked her profusely and immediately sent a retraction to the eleven DMV employees I had initially sent the email to. Problem solved.

That was that—so I thought.

Friday was here. It was the eve of a great weekend. I participated in a friend's wedding at Sacramento's McKinley Park Rose Garden on Saturday. I attended a circus at Arco Arena on Sunday. When Monday came around and it was time to return to work, the Klingerman Foundation email hoax was the furthest thing from my mind.

Then came the next day—Tuesday, September 11, 2001!

Shocked and horrified and traumatized at seeing what millions of others saw on TV, I emotionally pulled it together. I went to work at DMV's Media Relations Office on the top floor of the Department's 24th and Broadway (Building East) location.

We expected to receive a lot of press calls that day, but we didn't. DMV Management sent us home early.

The next day, DMV's Media Relations Office received calls. Callers asked to speak to Ron Owens. The eleven

DMV employees who initially received my Klingerman Foundation email, resent that email to other recipients. And then they resent it to more recipients and exponentially to more!

Because of what happened at the World Trade Center in New York, the Pentagon in Arlington, Virginia, and a field near Shanksville, Pennsylvania, curious reporters and worried people called DMV's Media Relations Office.

They asked whether the Klingerman Foundation blue envelope was laced with a toxic white powder.

Did twenty-three people get contaminated, sick, and die?

The warning must have been credible because "Ron Owens, Public Information Officer, Department of Motor Vehicles" and his phone number and his email address contained in the signature block displayed on the bottom made the Klingerman Foundation email that more credible.

Callers throughout California and the Midwest and east and even south in Florida called and asked to speak to Ron Owens.

Even a caller from London, England, called DMV's Media Relations Office and asked to speak to Ron Owens.

"Ron Owens is a straight-up guy," retired DMV Chief Deputy Director told me what he said to a Seattle friend after his friend received my Klingerman Foundation email. "If Ron Owens sent out that email, it must be true!"

True? Heavens no! It was NOT true!

I explained to many, many worried and concerned people. Most understood that I was victimized by a hoax, but a few got on my case.

One angry soldier from the Midwest chastised me for purposely preying on people's fears during 9/11. "I am going to come over there and kick your ass," he said.

"Ron, you are an honest man, and I highly respect you," my boss reassured me.

Yes, I am an honest man, but how could I have been dishonest? How could I have hidden that Klingerman Foundation virus callers were ringing the DMV Media Relations Office phone off the hook outside my boss's office door?

I informed DMV Chief Deputy Director. I confessed to DMV Director. I told them both while sitting in the Director's Suite what happened. I told them I was embarrassed. I told them I was ashamed. I literally felt this knot in the pit of my stomach because of the 9/11 shock, horror, and trauma we all collectively felt, which was exacerbated by the Klingerman Foundation hoax that I unwittingly perpetuated.

I am a Public Information Officer charged with communicating accurate information to the public. But in the days after the nation suffered the most horrific act of terrorism in history and in the days when we all thought terrorists would strike again; I, a DMV Public Information Officer, was causing people's fear, not allaying people's fear.

DMV's Media Relations Office received so many calls we had to develop an action plan.

So I drafted a holding statement indicating that the pathogen on the Klingerman Foundation envelope was a hoax. One of DMV's investigators assigned to help me manage this public information, public relations, and public education nightmare I caused reviewed that statement. We got approval from my superiors.

From that point moving forward, every time I received a Klingerman Foundation email query, I emailed that statement.

Meanwhile, DMV's IT shop closed my email address, changed a character in my name, and assigned me another email address. We finally handled the misinformation I caused.

It was I, a DMV Information Officer 1, who learned to question, research, and ascertain the veracity of information sent from a credible and trusted governmental official before believing it to be true. This 2001 hard lesson would bode well for me more than twenty years later.

CHAPTER 2
Questioned Flu Shots and Childhood Vaccines

It was I, a California Department Public Health (CDPH) Information Officer 2, who questioned the efficacy of flu shots and learned about the risks associated with childhood vaccines.

Years before March 2, 2009, when I walked in the sliding glass doors at 16th and Capitol Building in downtown Sacramento and embarked on what would be the start of my nearly fifteen-year CDPH career, I always thought that injecting the flu and inducing the flu to prevent the flu seemed illogical.

Yes, there is no "Dr." professional title preceding my name. There's no "MD" or "MPH" or "PhD" appearing after my name displayed on the back cover or inside this book. I am not an epidemiologist or an immunologist. I've never worn scrubs or donned a white physician's coat. I've never draped a stethoscope over my neck and made rounds in a hospital. I've never authored peer-reviewed articles published in prestigious medical journals. I respect those men and women who are medical professionals.

But in my common-sense layperson's opinion, I always struggled with the question of why anyone should ever inject themselves with the flu to fight the flu. It just never made sense to me. "What about home remedies and the holistic approach?" I'd ask myself.

I realize I am committing public health apostasy, but I never took a flu shot. I remember the-then Office of Public Affairs (OPA) Assistant Deputy Director chided me for not taking the flu shot after he inquired whether I injected myself. Assistant Deputy Director said I needed to get the flu shot to protect my elders. At that time, my parents were in their seventies, and my maternal grandmother had just turned one hundred years old. The four of us lived under one roof, and Assistant Deputy Director knew about my living situation. I stood quietly in the elevator after Assistant Deputy Director chided me, thinking that my elders didn't believe in the efficacy of flu shots either. They wouldn't want me to get injected to protect them.

Encouraging Californians to get seasonal flu shots every year was handled by other OPA Public Information Officers. They developed messaging with Center for Infectious Diseases (CID) subject matter experts, wrote talking points, and coordinated radio and television interviews in Spanish as well as English.

But for the first eleven years I worked at CDPH as an Information Officer 2, CID was not my portfolio. So I never dealt with it.

In the process of time, I learned about childhood vaccines. I learned about mama bears and papa bears having to care for their vaccine-injured children and refusing to vaccinate their other children.

Again, in my common-sense layperson's opinion, it just didn't make sense or seem right for California children to take eighty shots the first eighteen years of their lives.

In my common-sense layperson's opinion, this strict, rigorous childhood immunization schedule was tantamount to adults medically torturing children. I often wanted to ask public health professionals who push childhood vaccines if they were willing to be needled more than eighty times—about four times a year—for the next eighteen years of their lives.

The Office of Public Affairs management assigned me to work with the Center for Environmental Health, Center for Family Health, Office of Health Equity, and Laboratory Field Services (now Center for Laboratory Sciences) program staff.

Throughout the years, I've worked with program staff in developing messaging, talking points, and interviews on hundreds of media inquiries—from food recalls, food safety, water quality, West Nile Virus, Valley fever, skilled nursing facilities and hospitals to shellfish safety, health equity, sexually transmitted infections, sexually transmitted diseases, maternal mortality, infant mortality, genetic disease screening, plus a lot more.

Befriending the parents of a vaccine injured child caused me to finally deal with it.

In 2015, I met a Facebook friend who lives in North Carolina. Her son Luke was in great health until he took the vaccine. Talking to my North Carolina friend throughout the years really opened my eyes. It caused me to be more attuned to and commiserate with the concerns of mama bears and papa bears whose children were vaccine injured, and how they were treated really bothered me.

I worked at the Department of Toxic Substances Control (DTSC) as a Public Participation Specialist (PPS) from 1994-1998. One of the tenets of being a DTSC PPS is not to dismiss community and stakeholder concerns regarding toxic remediation. We were trained as PPS' to acknowledge that everyone's concerns are legitimate and are to be respected and considered.

But from what I observed throughout the years, CDPH ignored vaccine-injured children and their parents. Those who opposed vaccines were viewed as a public relations problem and an impediment of CDPH executing its mandated childhood immunization agenda.

Some politicians, public health officials, and mainstream media mouthpieces particularly dismissed parents' concerns. They called them "anti-vaxers" and branded them as "vaccine-hesitant." They castigated them as "radical" and characterized them as being on the fringe. They labeled them "conspiracy theorists" and denounced them as "right-wing extremists." They negatively characterized them as Neanderthals who disbelieve science. "Homeschoolers" and "homeschooling" were pejorative terms.

The name-calling, disrespect, and dismissiveness was just not right. As a matter of fact, it was unkind, insensitive, and downright cruel.

It also didn't seem right that the pharmaceutical industry was not held liable to those who were injured by the vaccines they manufactured. If their product was so "safe and effective," why enjoy such legal immunity?

An anti-vaccine rally was held at the north steps of the State Capitol one late afternoon. I don't specifically remember the year, but it must have been post 2015, the year I connected with my North Carolina Facebook friend. I attended that rally incognito after work. If rally attendees had known that a staff member of the California Department of Public Health's press office was in attendance, I would have been loudly booed. I got close. I stood to the right of the speakers. I listened intently to parents' stories. I saw their vaccine-injured children. Some of them were sitting in wheelchairs. My heart went out to them.

I've never believed in my common-sense layperson's world in an all-size-fits disease prevention or disease treatment approach. We are all "fearfully and wonderfully made" (Ps. 139:14) complicated, sophisticated, and unique multicellular organisms. This one-size-fits-all vaccination approach (particularly the COVID-19 vaccine) has injured, handicapped, and resulted in the deaths of many people, including possibly a loved one, you'll learn in Chapter 7 of this book.

Having learned about how vaccines—particularly childhood vaccines injuring kids—I became more suspicious of our annual influenza prevention messaging, but I kept my opinions to myself. Remember? CID was not my portfolio.

However, when another state department promoted one of our Information Officers, and he departed CDPH, Assistant Deputy Director assigned me that former Information Officer's CID portfolio. With what I learned from parents caring for their vaccine injured children, with what I saw at the anti-vaccine rally, and with what I heard from my North Carolina friend, her husband, and family in caring for Luke, I just could not accept that CID assignment.

In retrospect, I guess I played the conscientious objector card. Throughout the years, conscientious objectors refused—on moral or religious grounds—to serve in the military or bear arms in war. I refused on moral and deeply religious grounds to promote CDPH's "vaccines are safe and effective" message. I would be lying, according to my Christian beliefs and my moral code. I didn't want to put myself in breaking the ninth "thou shalt not lie" of the Ten Commandments.

So, I shared with Assistant Deputy Director my concerns. He understood my position and accommodated me. Thank the LORD—he assigned CID to another coworker due to my moral misgivings.

I didn't broach this topic with him, but I've heard that people have been injured taking flu vaccines. Is this true? I don't know. But I wish CDPH would check this out. I also learned that people who annually take flu shots have a great chance of developing dementia when they get older. Is this also true? I don't know. But again, I wish CDPH would investigate.

If I had my way, I would create a CDPH section that would study whether "vaccines are safe and effective." I'd organize a listening tour so California's public health officials and pharmaceutical representatives and stakeholders could hear from the vaccine-injured and their families.

It was I, a California Department Public Health Information Officer 2, who never took the flu shot and commiserated with the vaccine injured.

CHAPTER 3
Luke's Story

It was I, Luke, who was a bright-eyed and energetic big baby boy when I was born to my parents, but my body changed after doctors and nurses needled me.

I arrived on April 18, 2012. I was just one ounce shy of ten pounds when I came into the world and brightened my parents' day. I officially weighed nine pounds and fifteen ounces.

Mommy and Daddy told me I was two feet long. Nurses called me "The Two-Footer."

"Here's 'The Two-Footer' I was telling you about," one nurse told another nurse when I was carried throughout the hospital.

Mommy and Daddy laughed when they heard the nurses say this about me. My parents were so proud of me. I was their perfect, big bundle of two-foot-long joy.

Usually, babies roll over around four months old, not me. I did the rollover while lying on my back. Since I was such a big baby, I was strong. I remember sitting up, pulling up, lifting my head up, and rolling over—all pretty early.

At five months old, Mema, my Mommy's mommy, held my tiny hands. I was lying on my back. Mema lifted me up. She guided me to stand. I love-bit her. I wouldn't let go of her finger. Mommy laughed while she shot a video of me love-biting Mema.

I got my outside strength from Daddy. I got my inside strength from Mommy. I love Daddy. He's big, strong, and gentle. I love Mommy; she's small, strong, and patient.

There really wasn't a need for tummy time. I didn't need to do what babies do to strengthen their neck muscles and lift their heads. My neck muscles were already strong to lift my head. Daddy and Mommy said that at six-months-old, I was able to lift my head and sit up without their help.

Daddy and Mommy work out. One day, they watched me try to join them. I scooted over to play with one of their workout toys. My soft toys were easy to handle. Their toys weren't. Those were the heaviest toys I had ever seen! I tried to pick up one of their exercise toys. Yeah, I was strong, but I wasn't that strong. But I was determined.

I wasn't walking yet. I wasn't able to stand on my own. You see, I was around ten or eleven months old. I had to figure this out. So, I placed one hand against the nightstand for support. I bent down. I picked the weight up with my other hand. I wasn't that much taller than that exercise toy. Yet, I balanced myself. I got good at it. I picked the weight up with both hands. I lifted the weight a little off the ground.

Mommy didn't know if she should rush to grab it from me or cheer me on. She did both. I did this so often they video-recorded me.

I crawled around six or seven months old. I walked one day after my first birthday. I was very curious. I was very observant. I noticed everything. I noticed everyone around me.

After learning to walk, I loved playing chase with my sister. I call her Sissy. She had been playing all by herself for four long years. Sissy's life must have been really, really boring without me. I came along to play chase together, and we played other games.

I loved learning new words. And when I was a baby, I liked to say "shoe" and "no" a lot. When I started to learn how to count, I'd say, "One, two . . ." and before I said, "Three," I'd laugh and laugh and laugh.

Then, suddenly—at about thirteen months old, it was hard for me to breathe with a closed mouth. I blew yucky stuff out of my nose. Mommy gave me medicine every day to make me feel better, and she took me to the doctor's office often.

One day, it was harder for me to learn new words. I couldn't say "shoe" or "no." I couldn't count "One" and "Two." I didn't laugh before I said, "Three."

It was harder for me to think. It was harder for me to notice everything and everyone around me. I stopped talking. I'd stare off into space. I no longer looked at Mommy and Daddy in their eyes. I didn't want to play tag or play other games with Sissy. I didn't respond to my parents calling my name.

My eating changed. I didn't want to eat tasty meat, colorful fruit, or healthy vegetables. I wanted to eat food that came from boxes and packages.

I began to spin in circles and flap my hands. I was more sensitive and emotional. I'd make noises instead of talking. I ran and jumped. I pulled and pushed. I'd hit things when I got frustrated and angry.

My body didn't feel right. It was hard to think. It was if I was trapped in my body, and I couldn't tell Mommy and Daddy what was going on inside me.

It's been a long road. It takes me effort to do things other kids easily do—like running bath water and turning off knob, brushing teeth and rinsing mouth, dressing myself and picking up clothes, pushing feet in shoes and tying shoe strings, using fork and holding spoon, holding cup and drinking without straw, and writing my name and reading from memory.

I might not be able to tell you what day it is or how old I am all the time. I might not be able to tell you what month it is or my home address. I might not be able to say my name, Daddy's name, Mommy's name, Sissy's name, Mema's name, Papa's name. I might not be able to say the names of other family members. But I see their smiles. I feel their hugs. I feel the love of my family. I love my Mommy. I love my Daddy. I love Sissy. I love when they hold my hand. They understand me. They love me, and I love them.

I am not alone. Many children haven't been the same since we were needled. Many children have died after being needled.

Mommy shares my story to people she talks to on her phone. She shares my story with people she meets. Some people listen to her and are nice to her. Other people do not listen to her and are mean to her. But Mommy never stops.

She shared my story with Uncle Ron. He lives far away. He has sung a happy birthday song to me. He put me in his book.

I am now eleven. Mommy says God is fixing what they broke. Mommy says God is redoing what they did. Mommy says God is restoring the life doctors took from me.

Before she went to heaven, Uncle Ron's Mommy told my Mommy that I will become a doctor just like Luke in the *Bible*. When I am a doctor, I will help other needled kids.

It was I, Luke, who started to change and not feel like I felt when doctors and nurses pushed needles in my arm.

CHAPTER 4
Questioned COVID-19 Health Policies

It was I, an eleven-year California Department of Public Health (CDPH) employee at the time the pandemic came, who questioned health officials' response to COVID-19 and refused to comply with state directives and local mandates.

Learning about the risks associated with childhood vaccines and inwardly questioning the efficacy of flu shots caused me to be suspicious about whether face masks were effective in fighting COVID-19.

I was also skeptical about whether social distancing and teleworking—working from home—were also necessary.

When the COVID-19 pandemic in early 2020 came, I was never convinced that it was that serious for federal, state, and local mandates to lock everybody down and incarcerate everybody in their homes. I was never convinced that Mom-and-Pop stores had to be closed to prevent people from congregating in small areas, yet keep Target, Walmart, Sam's Club, and Costco Big-box stores open and people congregated in large areas.

I've known several Mom-and-Pop restaurants who are now closed. I'm sure you do too. Where I used to dine in downtown Sacramento, Mom-and-Pop eateries are all shuttered, from the Hungarian cuisine restaurant on J Street and eatery where I bought large chocolate chip cookies on K Street to the Chinese restaurant on L Street and the sandwich shop near Capitol Mall. These four businesses—and a plethora more—were all destroyed.

Good for corporate restaurants and good for their employees who survived the pandemic. But what about Mom-and-Pop businesses? The policies of the California Department of Public Health and the mandates of local health departments during the COVID-19 pandemic put a lot of people out of business or impeded their businesses.

When the COVID-19 pandemic came in early 2020, I was never convinced that we all needed to strap on blue paper masks. My ancestors were enslaved by iron manacles during slavery. Me and mine and you and yours and theirs and others were enslaved by blue paper masks during the pandemic. It doesn't matter if one was black and the other blue. It doesn't matter if one was iron and the other was paper, plastic, cloth, or other fabric. It doesn't matter if one was heavy and the other was light. I was convinced both were and are instruments of government-sanctioned submission and enslavement.

When the COVID-19 pandemic came in early 2020, my intellectual guard was up. We were told that we needed to put on a face mask when we walked away from our cubicles at work. But I walked around the seventh floor at the California Department of Public Health unmasked. I smiled at people (I'm a people person anyway). I waved at people down the long hallway. It was great seeing someone on the seventh floor. There weren't too many people who came to the building, so when someone did come to work, it was great seeing a familiar face.

I remember poking my head in the Center For Family Health's Assistant Deputy Director's office one day. She told me to stay at the doorway because I didn't have a face mask on. I respectfully complied to her wish and stayed at a distance.

I remember hearing a knock on the Office of Public Affairs door one day. I hurriedly got up from my cubicle seat. I briskly walked over to open the door. The current Office of Communications Deputy Director, who, at that time, was on loan to CDPH from the California Department of Developmental Services, asked me where my face mask was.

"I don't have one," I answered.

"Back up, sir," she retorted.

I respectfully complied and backed up.

During the late spring of 2020, temperatures began to increase in Sacramento. From my layperson's perspective, people wearing face masks at one-hundred-degree heat is dangerous.

So, I went to the Assistant Deputy Director's office and mentioned that it needed to be addressed, especially when temperatures increase. Sacramento temperatures are known to get to 105 to 110 degrees.

"Wouldn't it be dangerous for people to walk outside wearing a face mask in that kind of heat?" I asked Assistant Deputy Director while he sat and looked at his desktop computer.

I don't remember what he specifically said because he barked at me. He was under pressure, and I didn't take it personal. It was like he didn't want to hear it.

Perhaps he did not want to listen to me because maybe he agreed with me, but as a gubernatorial political appointee, he had to go along with Gov. Gavin Newsom's masking measures. Perhaps he did not want to hear me because at the time, he was preoccupied with writing an email. Perhaps he did not want to hear me because he knew I didn't agree with it, and he didn't want to hear my perspective.

I don't know. I just don't know.

During this time, it was unfortunate not seeing people smile. It was unfortunate not hearing people talk. It was unfortunate not viewing people's faces. Unfortunately, I grew accustomed to viewing foreheads and focusing on eyes. My heart went out to fast food employees, grocery store checkers, and restaurant waiters. They wore face masks day in and day out and night in and night out.

Face masks were problematic and impeded interpersonal communication and all of us from conducting interpersonal relationships. I know I am not alone by stating that I had difficulty hearing and problems understanding words uttered from masked mouths. Masks mask lips. Masks mask smiles. Masks mute voices. Masks suppress breath. Masks restrict breathing. Masks cause shortness of breath, lightheadedness, and forgetfulness. It is unknown the myriad of ailments, sickness, and diseases that may have developed among those who continually wore masks for a prolonged period of time.

I remembered sitting at my cubicle, and Assistant Deputy Director came over to my cubicle because I couldn't do something on my computer one day. He put a face mask on while I sat there at my computer—not wearing a face mask. I heard him ventilate. My heart went out to him; it really did.

"You don't have to wear a face mask around me," I thought and almost spoke.

But I kept my mouth shut to avoid an uncomfortable conversation.

If I had said anything, he would have argued about the efficacy of face masks, and I would have countered that wearing masks is like trying to stop a mosquito from flying through a chain link fence, Dr. Ramin Oskoui, a Washington D.C. cardiologist, told Fox News viewers on July 5, 2020. [6]

"There's no evidence that aerosolization of the virus is really a major transmitter," Oskoui explained on Fox News' Ingraham Angle that evening. "I think that it's very clear, and we've known this since February with the Crown Princess [cruise ship], that it's oral fecal spray —very much like polio or norovirus, and that's where aggressive hand-washing really plays a role.

"You also didn't mention the CDC guidance for May 20 of this year, that quotes other randomized control studies, some of which you reference, that simply show that masks for influenza like illnesses simply aren't effective.

"It's simple. Does your chain link fence stop a mosquito? It doesn't. That's, that's I think, the fundamental problem, and there's good randomized controlled data

---

[6] "Does your chain link fence stop a mosquito" July 15, 2020 Ronald F. Owens Jr Facebook post.

that suggests that the masks outside a strict medical setting simply don't slow transmission for viruses like Coronavirus."

Wouldn't it be great if CDPH reviewed this "good randomized controlled data" which Dr. Oskoui noted? Wouldn't it be great if CDPH studied the long-term health effects of continued masking?

During the long hot summer of 2020, it was sad to see people suffer. I heard one slim man audibly ventilate wearing a face mask. I saw a second man noisily breathe wearing a face mask. I witnessed a heavy-set man barely walk wearing a face mask. I saw countless people wear face masks outside in scorching ninety to one-hundred-degree heat! I've seen people wear saturated face masks in pouring rain! I've witnessed people adjust string wrapped around their ears. I saw people repeatedly touch and adjust face covers with unwashed hands. They endured their own breath condensate the lenses of their glasses. Foggy glass obfuscated their vision. I even saw a double-masked man sit in the car all by himself with his windows rolled up! And I spotted a helmeted motorcycle rider in oncoming traffic riding at freeway speed with his face shield lowered wearing a blue face mask. A Department of Motor Vehicles field office security guard loudly commanded me to remove my thick motorcycle helmet so I could put on a thin blue paper face mask; you'll read about it in Chapter 10.

I remember asking these questions then, and I ask these questions now: What about squinting eyes and perspired heads? What about hearts, brains, and lungs? What about oral hygiene? What about the possibility—indeed probability of infecting mouths and lips? What about epidermal discomfort? What about irritation caused by cloth, paper-like, or plastic material face masks touching and rubbing and scrapping against skin for a prolonged period of time?

These and more questions should be asked and investigated by a CDPH section that studies the long-term health effects of continued masking.

So when the COVID-19 pandemic came in early 2020 and everybody else teleworked at home, I was content coming to the office with a couple of coworkers. They seemed to be content coming to the office as well. One coworker worked part-time at home. The other coworker worked full time in the office.

It seemed like we were the only three CDPH employees who worked on the seventh floor. We liked coming to work. We're all old school anyway. We're used to getting up, getting ready, and commuting from suburbia to downtown as we had done years before.

One day, I was walking around Capitol Park—like I used to do before the pandemic—trying to stay fit and keep healthy by being outside. This was October 2020.

I came up to the left side of the building across the street from where I work. A man who carried two boxes had just exited that glass sliding door of that building. I could tell he was carrying two laptop computers inside them.

"Where are you taking these computers?" I asked with curiosity.

"Oh, I'm taking this across the street," the face-masked IT (information technology) man answered as we walked toward CDPH's 16th and Capitol Building.

We entered the lobby. We both brandished our badges to security. We strolled to the elevators, just feet away from security's front desk. I slightly leaned down and depressed the elevator button for him. The doors instantly opened. He walked inside. I followed him.

I instinctively depressed the seventh-floor button and asked him: "What floor?"

"Seven," IT Man said.

Since there seemed to be no one in the building, we quickly ascended nonstop to the seventh floor. Upon arriving at our destination, I clearly expected IT Man to turn left, walk down the hallway, and pivot right, heading to the Director's Suite. Instead, he turned right where I was heading.

"I've got my key," I said, holding my credit card resembling a CDPH ID magnetic key. "I'll unlock the door for you."

I heard the door unlock and opened it for IT Man. He walked inside the Office of Public Affairs (OPA). The OPA Administrative Assistant was sitting at her front desk. Administrative Assistant normally didn't come into the office, but an arrangement had apparently been previously made to meet with IT Man.

"These two computers are for Ron and (won't divulge coworker's name)," IT Man said.

"There must be another Ron who works here," I thought, aware that OPA staff had grown because of contractors, loaned employees from other state agencies, and new staff.

"This is for you, Ron," Administrative Assistant reiterated.

"They issued me a laptop," I thought, thinking that I was tacitly being told to telework.

It was like Christmas in October because I received a state-issued laptop computer, power cord, and mouse.

"Well, I'll have to take it home and try it out," I told IT Man and Administrative Assistant.

After work, I took my state-issued laptop home. Shortly thereafter, I called OPA's Assistant Deputy Director.

"Hey," I remember saying gleefully. "It works. I'm able to log on to my home Wi-Fi, so I'm good to go."

I asked Assistant Deputy Director to telework one day. I was pleasantly surprised that I had no technological issues working remotely. I proposed teleworking regularly—like on Tuesdays and Thursdays.

"That'd be fine," I heard Assistant Deputy Director say to me over my iPhone.

Between October and mid-December 2020, I commuted downtown and worked in the office on Mondays, Wednesdays, and Fridays. I stayed at home and teleworked on Tuesdays and Thursdays.

However, a terminal family situation altered my telework schedule. In mid-December, my mother, Dora L. Owens, was told by her oncologist that she had six months to live. I had a serious conversation with Assistant Deputy Director that cold and dark Friday evening.

"I'd like to telework full time so I can take care of my mother," I stated to Assistant Deputy Director.

"Of course," he said without hesitation.

From mid-December 2020 to June 13, 2021, when my mother passed, I worked at home. It was a blessing to work at home yet still attend to her as well and attend to my dad. (It's well into 2023, and I still telework. I had to admittedly be dragged—kicking and screaming to telework.)

CDPH leadership seems to be fine with many staff members never working in the building. They have encouraged people to stay at home. As a matter of fact, our staff grew from about ten to twelve people when I first walked in the door on March 2, 2009. With all the permanent employees and contractors, the Office of Communications has hired, at the writing of this book in September 2023, more than thirty-five coworkers.

If we all wanted to work on the seventh floor of the building, there wouldn't be any room for all of us. I don't know how the powers that be plan to address that issue in the months and years to come. Just like I wasn't privy to knowing who decided to issue my coworker and me a laptop computer, I am not privy to knowing how the department will address teleworking versus working on-site.

During the first nine months of the pandemic, I walked around the seventh floor—the same floor as the Directorate—where California's public health policy is promulgated. I walked around there without a face mask.

When the COVID-19 pandemic came in early 2020, my job was not even to handle any COVID-19 media requests. They were content with my coworker and I responding to non-COVID-19 media requests. And that's what we did. I didn't have to deal with the rollout of COVID-19 vaccines.

After my mother died and was buried and while the COVID-19 pandemic ensued, I managed my grief accordingly and started watching what was going on around me. I began to scrutinize more because I was assigned to copy reporter names, their media outlets, email addresses, phone numbers, and questions from the Office of Public Affairs' email in basket and paste all that information— plus indicate the assigned Public Information Officer— into a Word file.

I was given that mundane record keeping assignment in October 2021. I did that daily assignment through May 2023.

As a team player, I didn't mind in the least doing that kind of grunt yet important work. But with all due respect, this was a job for a student intern, not a seasoned Information Officer 2 who was told from an anonymous reliable source months earlier that the Newsom Administration was considering me to serve as a Deputy Director in the comms shop at another state agency. I wouldn't have pursued or accepted such a gubernatorial political appointment anyway because I am ideologically opposed to Gov. Newsom, but my point is that I was way over qualified to do what I was tasked to do.

It was I, a California Department Public Health employee, who commiserated with small businesses, never covered my face, teleworked to care for my mother and was not assigned any COVID-19 vaccination media inquiries.

CHAPTER 5
My Ivermectin Email

It was he, Center for Environmental Health Deputy Director, who asked three Office of Communications staff members to comment on a California Department of Public Health (CDPH) website advisory draft that addressed the misuse of ivermectin to treat COVID-19.

CEH Deputy Director solicited, in an October 6, 2021, email, the opinions of the Office of Communications Deputy Director, Assistant Deputy Director, and Information Officer 2 (me). I had been assigned to work with CEH program staff years earlier, and because of that managerial assignment, I was very familiar with CEH programs and its subject matter experts.

CEH Deputy Director addressed in that Wednesday email to we three "Comms folks" that CDPH's advisory was to provide specific warnings and information for consumers and health care providers from CEH's Food and Drug Branch (FDB), based on the Centers for Disease Control and Prevention health advisory.

CEH Deputy Director provided additional context in his email.

"In response to ongoing media attention regarding the unapproved use of human and veterinary ivermectin products for the treatment of COVID-19, it is important to provide accurate and easily accessible guidance to combat the dangerous misinformation surrounding such uses," he wrote.

"The unapproved use of ivermectin has placed an increased burden on poison control centers, resulted in multiple cases of toxicity nationwide, and created a shortage of veterinary ivermectin products," he further wrote. "Educating the public via multiple means is important to protect human health, prevent product shortages, and encourage individuals to consult with their doctor for the prevention and treatment of COVID-19."

CEH Deputy Director indicated that the plan was to post CDPH's advisory on FDB's website on Friday, October 8.

"It [CDPH's advisory] will be ADA compliant," he assured us. "Please let us know if there are any concerns or other feedback."

CDPH's Director and Assistant Director, CEH's Assistant Deputy Director and Assistant Division Chief, plus two Assistant Governmental Program Analysts were copied in his email.

I remember sitting in my chair, staring at the screen of my silver state-issued laptop in paralyzed shock. I couldn't believe CEH Deputy Director was so dismissive of ivermectin, while pondering over the email. "What a great opportunity for me to respond," I thought because he wanted my two bosses and I to weigh in on a statement that was going to be published on CDPH's website warning Californians about the dangers of ivermectin.

At that time, I had been listening to several very credible peer-reviewed medical subject matter experts on several podcasts who, in my common-sense layperson's observation, are far more experienced than CDPH officials. These physicians, who had actually treated COVID-19 patients months before and CDPH officials had not, were telling us that, yes, Yes, YES—properly dosed ivermectin could cure COVID-19!

When I received CEH Deputy Director's email, I could not sit and let that go, especially since he asked my two bosses and me to "let us know if there are any concerns or other feedback." Furthermore, one of my man codes is stated in Proverbs 3:27: "Withhold not good from them to whom it is due, when it is in the power of thine hand to do it." It would have been morally reprehensible if I had withheld good information that could help 40 million Californians.

Plus, I was asked, amongst others who were my superiors, to opine on what he was going to do. It would have been cowardly and morally vapid of me not to respond by providing information from physicians who had treated COVID-19 patients.

Remember when I was a Department of Motor Vehicles Media Relations Office staffer, and a known, credible, and trusted government source forwarded me that Klingerman Foundation email, and it turned out to be untrue? Well, I learned from that hard experience more than twenty years earlier to ascertain the veracity of information sent from a trusted governmental official— in this instance CEH Deputy Director— before believing it.

And who has more weight, credible peer-reviewed subject matter experts who treated and cured thousands of COVID-19 patients with ivermectin or CEH Deputy Director who outright denounced ivermectin?

I conducted research. I pulled information and facts together. I figured I had one time to get it right. So I solicited the opinions and advice of several people—I called them my council of elders who I greatly respect. That council of elders were the Deputy Press Secretary of a large state department and retired Deputy Director of Communications from another major state department, a discovery attorney who practices law on the East Coast, a couple of other close friends whose spiritual insight I cherish, and Peter A. Baldridge, a retired public health attorney. Peter wrote the Foreword in this book.

In 2007, he wrote the regulations metamorphosing the Department of Health Services into the California Department of Public Health. Peter was also CDPH's Assistant Chief Counsel from 2009–2014.

It took me about five days to write my draft. At that time, it was the most important email I had ever drafted in my then-twenty-seven-year state service career. My council of elders reviewed it. They opined on it. They edited it.

And after all that, yes, I prayed on it.

Thus, at 9:16 pm on October 13, 2021, I replied all. I sent my email to CEH Deputy Director and Office of Comms Assistant Deputy Director.

I copied CDPH's Director and Assistant Director, Office of Comms Deputy Director, CEH's Assistant Deputy Director and Assistant Division Chief, and two rank-and-file Assistant Governmental Program Analysts (AGPA)— one AGPA from the Directorate and the other with CEH.

The tone of my email was buoyant and optimistic. I wanted to be hopeful. I opened that I wanted to share some great news, just in case CDPH received media coverage about this topic. I stated that Dr. Pierre Kory, a lung and ICU specialist, said more than 8,000 COVID-19 patients had been successfully treated with ivermectin. I provided the link of Dr. Kory's sixteen-page "Homeland Security Committee Meeting: Focus on Early Treatment of COVID-19." I stated that in his US Senate testimony, he provided data "supporting ivermectin as a potential global solution to the COVID-19 pandemic." [7]

I provided background. I noted that late last year (2020), Dr. Kory summarized existing clinical studies in the prevention (over 2,400 patients), early treatment (over 3,000), and late treatment (approached 3,000) phases of COVID-19.

"Nearly all studies are demonstrating the therapeutic potency and safety of ivermectin in preventing transmission and progression of illness in nearly all who take this drug," Dr. Kory testified before the US Senate's Homeland Security Committee on December 8, 2020.

It was important for me to provide information indicating Dr. Kory's credibility. So I wrote that he was the former Chief of the Critical Care Service and Medical Director of the Trauma and Life Support Center at the University of Wisconsin. I wrote how Dr. Kory said that ivermectin "is highly safe, widely available, and low cost" in the treatment of COVID-19.

"I have seen so many vibrant fathers and mothers of families die in my ICU," said Dr. Kory, who led ICU's and personally treated over 100 hospitalized COVID-19 patients in New York City, Greenville, South Carolina

---

[7] Dr. Pierre Kory, "Testimony of Pierre Kory, MD, Homeland Security Committee Meeting: Focus on Early Treatment of COVID-19," US Senate Homeland Security Committee, December 8, 2020.

and Milwaukee, Wisconsin. "And most importantly, the majority are minorities, Black and Latinos—many of them poor and often without access to private doctors for early treatment. I have never seen such a disparity in any other illness I treat."

I noted in my email that I cared deeply for all humanity, but as a Black man, Dr. Kory's statement really resonated with me.

I informed email recipients that Dr. Kory is the president of Front Line COVID-19 Critical Care Alliance" (FLCCC), "a 501(c)(3) non-profit organization dedicated to developing highly effective treatment protocols to prevent the transmission of COVID-19 and to improve the outcomes for patients ill with the disease." [8]

He and six other physicians founded FLCCC in March 2020. I embedded an FLCCC link for them to read more about COVID-19 critical care. I also embedded another link that has Dr. Kory's bio, as well as the bios of his other colleagues, which includes all of their curriculum vitae.

When citing a list of "Dr.," it is journalistically customary, for brevity and to avoid redundancy, to use "Dr." only once, such as Drs. Paul E. Marik, Flávio A. Cadegiani, Joseph Varon, Jose Iglesias, Keith Berkowitz, and Fred Wagshul.

However, I wanted to make a point before CDPH's senior leadership. I wanted them to read "Dr." preceding each and every name. So I repeatedly cited "Dr.," that is, Dr. Paul E. Marik, Dr. Flávio A. Cadegiani, Dr. Joseph Varon, Dr. Jose Iglesias, Dr. Keith Berkowitz, and Dr.

---

[8] Google Front-Line COVID-19 Critical Care Alliance.

Fred Wagshul, to rhythmically punctuate individual as well group credibility of these six physicians.

I embedded a link of an October 7, 2021, Dr. Kory tweet. In that tweet, he wrote,"Between 100-200 United States Congress Members (plus many of their staffers & family members) with COVID were treated by a colleague over the past 15 months with ivermectin & the I-MASK+protocol at flccc.net [https://covid19critical-care.com/] none have gone to the hospital. Just sayn'."

Responding to those who asked him "for sources/names," Dr. Kory subsequently tweeted that "1) this came from a highly credible source inside Congress who has asked to remain anonymous" and 2) "I would never divulge the medical treatments of individual members, nor do I know them myself."

"I fully stand by this tweet," he concluded.

As I reflect at the time of writing this chapter of this book—I'm nearing the two-year anniversary of my ivermectin email—I get riled when I think about the hypocrisy. It was and still is unbelievable to me that members of Congress and their staff and their families were taking ivermectin privately, yet these same Congress members were either badmouthing ivermectin publicly or refused to say ivermectin works. Just think of the lives they could have saved had they only told the masses that properly dosed ivermectin cures COVID-19!

In my October 13, 2021, email, I shared that perhaps our subject matter experts can reach out to Dr. Kory and his FLCCC colleagues.

I stated, "In accordance with performing my essential function as a CDPH Information Officer II, which is to advise 'department staff of the public relations implications of department policy decisions,' I want to provide you all this heads up just in case CDPH is scrutinized and receives media coverage about this topic."

I also noted that I viewed my research and writing this email as an essential function of being an Information Officer 2.

"But most importantly," I stressed, "in addition to warning people against using veterinarian ivermectin, CDPH has an even greater opportunity to take the national lead—indeed the international lead—in saving lives by investigating or advocating for the use of properly dosed ivermectin by the medical community. It would behoove CDPH to look at therapeutic treatment, such as ivermectin."

I acknowledged in my email that it took a while for me to respond, especially since—I implied but didn't explicitly state—CEH Deputy Director initially noted that the plan was to post CDPH's advisory on the Food and Drug Branch's website on Friday, October 8.

"In closing, it's been a week and I want to apologize for just now responding," I wrote. "This is probably the most important email I've sent in my 27-year career in California state service. Sending you this important information required a great deal of preparation; it required time to carefully research, read, and process Dr. Kory's DHS testimony. Additionally, drafting this email necessitated mentation, an additional investment of time and critical reflection."

I continued. "In this time when so many Americans have lost loved ones, friends and coworkers, I reflect on the loss of my own 89-year-old mother on June 13, 2021. While she didn't succumb to COVID-19, her death from multiple myeloma—a cancer of plasma cells—causes me to empathize with the survivors whose loved ones died from COVID-19. It is my hope that by this careful review of this research and information we may be able to save countless lives, not only in the United States but throughout the world."

I thanked them for their time and careful consideration.

I purposely played several cards. I purposely played the magnanimous card (stating we have a great opportunity for the California Department of Public Health to take the statewide, national, and international lead). I purposely played the race card (being politically correct in front of ideological liberals who espouse diversity, equity, and inclusion). I purposely played the California Department of Public Health Information Officer 2 card (citing that I'm doing my job). I purposefully played the twenty-seven-year state service card (indicating I'm a seasoned employee). And yes, I purposely and genuinely played the sympathy card (my late mother died four months earlier).

What was the purpose of me playing all these cards? Well, it's not for this audience (CDPH staff). My email could be seen by anyone who files a California Public Records Act request in the future. My email could be seen by the Bureau of State Audits (should CDPH brass retaliate against me), lawyer(s), court(s), judge(s), mainstream media, alternative media, and so on.

But at the time I drafted that email, I never envisioned in my wildest imagination that all of this information would actually be published in a book, titled *Muzzled Truth*.

I had to cover my bases, purposefully play all those cards on the table for all to see in one document, and protect myself and my father, Ronald F. Owens Sr.

I didn't know what they might do to me, especially since the Office of Public Affairs (OPA) Deputy Director wrote me up four years earlier the first time she held the Deputy Director position. The reason why OPA Deputy Director wrote me up in 2017 was because I did not see a couple of Public Record Act (PRA) request emails in my basket, and I missed the PRA-mandated ten-day response deadline. Yes, she was managerially justified to do so. However, if Gov. Jerry Brown had just promoted me to be his Deputy Press Secretary, and I was just about to walk out the door to work in a high-ranking visible position in the Brown Administration, I would have afforded grace to the subordinate at my existing shop. I would have pulled subordinate aside, inquired what was going on in his or her life that affected job performance—I was still mourning the death of my late 106-year-old maternal grandmother—and offered verbal correction. However, OPA Deputy Director didn't or doesn't manage that way.

We have daily 9:45 a.m. and 10:00 a.m. teleconference staff meetings via our state-issued laptops. The meeting that occurred the day after I sent my ivermectin email lasted for only four minutes. I believe that was the shortest meeting ever. Office of Comms Assistant Deputy Director, my then-immediate supervisor, presided over that meeting. Deputy Director wasn't able to join, which is not unusual. Assistant Deputy Director said Deputy Director was in another meeting. The staff usually shares a quote of the day. We didn't that day. I sensed that my ivermectin email sent shockwaves throughout the department. I wondered if Deputy Director was conferring with the powers that be about it. I don't know this for certain, but this is what I sensed.I sure would like to have read reactionary emails and eavesdropped on conversations that probably occurred.

On Thursday, October 14, 2021, Assistant Deputy Director, who was my immediate supervisor, emailed me at 5:45 pm. This is what he wrote.

> Good evening, Ron:
>
> We don't have an issue with you providing a heads up or sharing information. However, before reaching out to CDPH leadership, please run all information pertaining to the fight against COVID-19, or another health topic by [Deputy Director first name] and I first so that we may consider the best way to proceed.
>
> The excerpt from your email (below) is not your area of expertise. Furthermore, California/CDPH/FDB does not approve the use of pharmaceuticals—that is under federal/FDA jurisdiction (and requires clinical trials, etc.).
>
> *But most importantly, in addition to warning people against using veterinarian ivermectin, CDPH has an even greater opportunity to take the national lead— indeed the international lead—in saving lives by investigating or advocating for the use of properly dosed ivermectin by the medical community. It would behoove CDPH to look at therapeutic treatment, such as ivermectin.*

Please let me know if you have any questions.

While writing this chapter of *Muzzled Truth*, I learned CDPH approved a new biomedical intervention to prevent sexually transmitted infections (STIs), according to an April 28, 2023, three-page letter sent to health care providers. If homosexuals and transgender women engage in condomless oral, anal, or vaginal sex and ingest the antibiotic doxycycline—when taken as doxy-PEP—chlamydia, gonorrhea, and syphilis is significantly reduced. So CDPH approved this pharmaceutical to prevent STIs, yet CDPH would not investigate the efficacy of ivermectin!

Dear Reader and Listener, do you get this? The California Department of Public Health is more focused on facilitating same-sex intercourse than using ivermectin to save lives from COVID-19!

I am disgusted! (Deep exhale.)

Assistant Deputy Director corrected me on how I should have responded to CEH Deputy Director's email, noted that I am not a subject matter expert and told me what CDPH can't do rather than indicating what CDPH can do to save lives.

It was he, Office of Public Affairs (OPA) Assistant Deputy Director, who instructed me to first apprise OPA management if I had concerns about CDPH's fight against the pandemic, stated the department's policy regarding not approving pharmaceuticals, and told me that I'm not a subject matter expert—after I provided information that properly dosed ivermectin can cure people of COVID-19.

CHAPTER 6
"Mindful Meditation"

It was he, California Department of Public Health (CDPH) Director, who conducted religious rituals on state time in front of state employees at the beginning of state meetings.

And it was I, an Information Office 2 and Supervisor, who was duty-bound to file two claims with CDPH's Civil Rights Unit (CRU) because the most powerful person of the department was exercising and imposing his religion in the Department.

I'm sharing this incident in this chapter of *Muzzled Truth* because this incident prepared and emboldened me to battle an inter-departmental information war that I did not know was coming. This "mindful meditation" incident steeled me to have the courage to tell CDPH management what a Biden Administration official shockingly said about COVID-19 vaccines four months later.

But four months earlier (December 9, 2021), CDPH Director conducted a "mindful meditation" session incident before hundreds of CDPH's employees during "CDPH's Virtual Holiday Open House."

Having taken the mandated "CDPH Workplace Harassment Prevention (Supervisors)" training days before—which taught supervisors to speak up when witnessing potential violations—I filed the first claim.

In my December 17, 2021, complaint, I noted that "mindful meditation" is rooted in Hinduism and Buddhism. I alleged that it's inappropriate for state employees to exercise religion in the workplace. I asserted that CDPH's Director should not have conducted one-minute meditative sessions. I indicated that the submission of this complaint is not intended to be inimical and that my complaint is just a friendly or gentle correction.

In my complaint, I also noted that this issue was easily soluble. I simply requested that CDPH Director refrain from practicing "mindful meditation" sessions during state time using state resources in front of state employees—out of respect for others who practice other religions and those who hold nonreligious beliefs.

CDPH Director continuing to conduct "mindful meditation," I further asserted, showed he was violating my faith and the faith of others. It showed a systematic pattern of him using the power of his directorship, abusing his power, and imposing his religious views on all of us.

However, after investigating, Equal Employment Opportunity Officer (EEOC) and Chief Internal Auditor Deputy Director determined that my complaint submitted to CRU did not meet a prima facie case of discrimination based on religion.

Interpreting CRU's conclusion, I think EEOC Deputy Director's point was that if I was prevented from singing a Christmas carol or prohibited from reading Scripture about the birth of Jesus Christ, yet CDPH Director was permitted to conduct "mindful meditation," then I would have had a case, resulting in a favorable outcome.

CRU indicated it would not take further action. CRU also indicated that the material gathered during the course of this investigation had been elevated to CDPH's leadership to discuss alternatives to address the information provided.

In other words, CDPH Director was probably (hopefully) notified of my complaint.

Therefore, CRU closed my religious discrimination complaint on January 26, 2022.

During his discussions about leadership, CDPH Director discussed meekness and leading with humility. CDPH Director stated that managers and supervisors needed to be able to admit they're wrong. Therefore, I really thought CDPH Director would not conduct any more "mindful meditations." I honestly thought that was that. However, I was gravely wrong.

On April 5, 2022, CDPH Director conducted a "Mindfulness Minute" session during CDPH's "State of Public Health Town Hall" virtual meeting.

"To get us started, we're going to go ahead and do a mindfulness minute," said CDPH Director before hundreds of employees.

I was shocked! I was aghast. I couldn't believe what I was hearing. CDPH Director was probably notified of my complaint, yet he still insisted on conducting "mindful meditation" anyway.

"So wherever you're at, just relax in your chair," said CDPH Director. "Gaze down or close your eyes, and just follow my instructions."

Take some slow deep breaths.

And I want you to focus on your breathing.

[26.58 seconds of meditative silence ensued.]

If you have a thought just acknowledge it and let it go.

You have a feeling just acknowledge and let it go.

[8.40 seconds of meditative silence transpired.]

So mindfulness is the awareness that arises by focusing on purpose --paying attention in the moment, without judgment or expectation.

[8.95 seconds of meditative silence proceeded.]

So you're focusing on your breathing, and feel how it makes your body feel. Just notice the sensations as you take slow deep breaths.

[23.55 seconds of more meditative silence]

So focusing on the present moment, without judgment or expectation.

[10.97 seconds of final meditative silence]

"Okay, why don't we go ahead and open your eyes and in future sessions," said CDPH Director, who proceeded with a detailed explanation.

I'll talk a little bit more about the neuro-science of mindfulness. Mindfulness is like riding on a treadmill, or going for a run, it makes your body stronger. So you think about right when you run on a tread-mill makes your body stronger, but that strength is with you, when you're doing other activities throughout the day.

It's the same thing with mindfulness. It makes your mind stronger, the ability to focus. And so that ability to focus helps you at other times, when you're just doing your work and interacting with people to —to be there to be present, to be present with folks.

"And the two words that I like that go along with that is kindness and curiosity is to be present with kindness and curiosity. And that'll really help you. So let's go to the next slide."

CDPH Director concluded and proceeded with his PowerPoint presentation.

Personally, I felt spiritually violated and disrespected when he proceeded with his "Mindfulness Minute" session that April 5, 2022, morning.

My biblical/Christian faith teaches to respect others, just as I imagine Hinduism and Buddhism teaches adherents. My biblical/Christian faith also teaches to meditate on the Word of God, not let thoughts and feelings go while meditating by "focusing on my breathing" or "focusing on the present moment." My biblical/Christian faith also teaches not to focus on ourselves but fixate our attention on Jesus Christ.

Even though EEOC Deputy Director elevated my concerns the previous January "to CDPH's leadership to discuss alternatives to address the information provided," CDPH's Director, the most powerful man in the department, still insisted on holding, during state time and using state resources, "Mindfulness Minute" session. He is imposing his religious beliefs on others.

My second complaint, as well as my first complaint, was spurred by me taking "CDPH Workplace Harassment Prevention (Supervisors)" mandated training the previous December, I told the California Department of Justice (DOJ) Deputy Attorney General, who interviewed me.

After filing a second complaint with CRU, EEOC Deputy Director outsourced my complaint to the California's DOJ.

I also told California DOJ Deputy Attorney General that this mandatory training instructs us to speak up when we witness potential violations. "It's just not only about me," I told DOJ Deputy Attorney General. It's about acknowledging the religious beliefs of others and respecting those who hold nonreligious beliefs.

The outcome for the second complaint was the same as the first complaint.

On July 5, 2022, EEOC Deputy Director, representing California's DOJ Deputy Attorney General, closed my complaint.

"Based on the information and documentation provided, the complaint does not meet that prima facie elements for a complaint of religious discrimination or harassment, nor did it rise to the level of a potential violation of CDPH policy," the official closure memorandum read. "Therefore, CRU would not take any further action."

I imagine if I was prohibited from praying in the name of Jesus before a CDPH staff meeting, yet CDPH Director was permitted to conduct "mindful meditation," then my complaint might have had merit and resulted in a favorable outcome.

I could have pressed the matter further. I could have exercised the option of filing a complaint with the Department of Fair Employment and Housing or the US Equal Employment Opportunity Commission. I could have even asked to pray at a staff meeting with the expectation of being denied just to make a point. But I would have been hypocritical. I would have been guilty of violating the same law or policy I had accused CDPH Director of violating.

It is he, California Department of Public Health's Director, who still conducts "mindful meditation" on state time in front of state employees at the beginning of state meetings, but he now says employees can opt out from participating.

And it was I, Ronald Owens, who did not know filing these two complaints prepared and emboldened me to inform CDPH leadership that COVID-19 vaccines are killing people.

CHAPTER 7

COVID-19 Vaccines "Are
Killing People..."

It was I, Ronald Owens, who emailed the California Department of Public Health (CDPH) leadership and notified them a Biden Administration health official said COVID-19 vaccines are killing people of color at about two times the rate of White Americans. [9]

But CDPH's Office of Communications management initially ignored me, subsequently threatened disciplinary action against me, rudely muzzled me, and, finally, gaslighted me.

It was the end of a trying and stressful week. I walked into the emergency room of Kaiser Permanente South Sacramento Medical Center on the evening of August 25, 2023. I had felt chest pains the past couple of days. The chest pains I felt then reminded me of the chest pains I felt on February 23, 2019. That was the day I was diagnosed with blood clots in both my lungs.

In addition, my left leg was swollen and felt tighter than usual that Friday evening. My left leg has actually

---

[9] "White House Convening on Equity," The White House's YouTube channel, last modified April 14, 2022.

been swollen for years. Kaiser previously diagnosed that swelling as deep vein thrombosis (DVT). I wondered if the DVT plus chest pains were connected to the February 2019 blood clots in both lungs incident more than four years earlier—hence, my concern. But the swelling in my left leg that August evening was more uncomfortable. In addition to my left leg tightness, it felt slightly feverish.

Because of what I witnessed and experienced at CDPH and what I observed elsewhere the past three years, I just didn't trust capitalistic corporate medicine, particularly Kaiser. No negative reflection on the hardworking men and women who serve patients there; I just don't trust the medical establishment.

On Thursday, a friend encouraged me to go to the doctor. Earlier that Friday, a coworker urged me to get myself checked out. So, I finally acquiesced to their advice.

Kaiser medical staff conducted an electrocardiogram, X-ray, and ultrasound. Throughout the evening, in between those tests, I reflected on the events that happened that week and transpired over the past couple of years.

You see, the day before (Thursday, August 24, 2023) my visit to Kaiser's emergency room, I wrote an email to the California Department of Public Health's Assistant Director. I copied CDPH's Office of Communications Deputy Director, Assistant Deputy Director, and Media Team Supervisor.

The text in the email subject line displayed: "Re: HHS Secretary Xavier Becerra's COVID-19 Vaccines 'Killing People…' Comment & Management's Retaliatory Actions for Me Reporting It."

I explained to CDPH Assistant Director that on April 14, 2022, the United States Department of Health and Human Services Secretary Xavier Becerra spoke at the White House's "Convening on Equity" virtual summit. At the 45:50 mark of the Official White House YouTube video streaming the summit, Secretary Becerra said the following:

> *"Secondly, by having better data, we can do a couple of things. Vaccines a year ago today, by the way, we know that vaccines are killing people of color, Blacks, Latinos, Indigenous People at about two times the rate of White Americans. So on vaccines last year, we saw that about two-thirds of White American adults had received at least one shot of vaccine . . ."*

When he said that, I could not believe it. I stopped, scrolled back the YouTube video, and repeatedly played that section over again. After watching and listening to several replays, I noticed Becerra didn't hesitate. He didn't fumble for words. He just outright said it. And he said it to two Black women. They didn't say, "Secretary Becerra, can you back that up? They didn't ask: "Did you misspeak?" They didn't state, "Would you like to clarify?" They just sat there!

I informed CDPH Assistant Director that I embedded the Official White House YouTube video link.[10] I directed to scroll to the 45:50 mark. I stated, to hear Secretary Becerra's response in context to the question asked of him, scroll back to the 42:53 mark of that video.

---

[10] Ibid.

I noted that I care deeply for all humanity, but as a Black man, what Secretary Becerra said: "we know that vaccines are killing people of color," resonated with me and deeply disturbed me.

I apprised CDPH Assistant Director the day before my Kaiser emergency room visit that on April 18, 2022, at 11:58 a.m., I sent an email to my two bosses, in accordance with Assistant Deputy Director, who told me six months earlier—as a response to my properly dosed ivermectin can cure COVID-19 email—to "please run all information pertaining to the fight against COVID-19, or another health topic by [Deputy Director name] and I first so that we may consider the best way to proceed." I informed CDPH Assistant Director that my April 18, 2022, email was sent to Office of Communications Deputy Director, and I copied Media Team Supervisor because Secretary Becerra's statement shocked, alarmed, and concerned me.

In that email I stated to CDPH Assistant Director, I informed Office of Public Affairs (OPA) management what Secretary Becerra said. I stated that CDPH had messaged and branded that COVID-19 vaccines "are safe and effective." I noted these vaccines have not been "safe and effective" for many people.

I reported that more than 1.25 million reports were filed, 26,976 people died, and thousands have been injured by COVID-19 vaccines, according to the Vaccine Adverse Events Reporting System (VAERS). I listed the number of hospitalizations (149,527), urgent care visitations (127,492) and doctor office visits (187,893). I listed the current number of the types of injuries people sustained.[11] And according to VAERS,[12] those injuries are anaphylaxis (9,615), Bell's palsy (15,110), miscarriages (4,496), heart attacks (13,819), myocarditis/pericarditis (38,605), permanently disabled (50,100), thrombocytopenia/low platelet (6,379), life-threatening (30,293), severe allergic reaction (41,556), and shingles (13,413).

I embedded that VAERS link and noted VAERS is co-managed by the US Centers for Disease Control and Prevention, which is under Secretary Becerra's Department of Health and Human Services.

I asked OPA Deputy Director on April 18, 2022, if it would be prudent if CDPH management, California Health and Human Services Agency officials, and Governor's Office personnel be made aware of Secretary Xavier Becerra's concerning comment and VAERS data.

I closed by sharing that a seventy-six-year-old close family member was in relatively good health, considering her age. She took the vaccine in March 2021. Her health rapidly declined. She was in and out of the hospital. Unable to take care of herself, she moved in with another closer relative. I stated that I was sad to report she died last July.

I acknowledged that we may never know whether the COVID-19 vaccine had anything to do with her rapid declining health and eventual death. But in light of Secretary Becerra's concerning comment and this alarming VAERS data, I wonder if my family member's death was indeed vaccine-related.

---

[11] Vaccine Adverse Events Reporting System (VAERS), co-managed by the Centers for Disease Control and Prevention's (CDC), as of April 8, 2022.

[12] Ibid.

Responding at 2:41 p.m. on that Monday, Deputy Director thanked me for my email and copied Media Team Supervisor.

I don't know if Deputy Director apprised her superiors. But every day that transpired from that point on weighed on me. Nevertheless, I suppressed my feelings and went along.

Time transpired. The weight of COVID-19 vaccine injuries and deaths weighed on me more. I checked VAERS data.

On October 13, 2022, at 4:54 p.m., I emailed Deputy Director a nearly six-month update. I noted that I was sad to report that there had been an increase of COVID-19 vaccine injuries and deaths, according to VAERS.

As of Monday, October 3, 2022,[13] I reported that 1,424,789 injury reports had been filed, and 31,330 people had been reported to have died from COVID-19 vaccines. (That's a 4,354 increase of people who died.) Again, I listed the current number of hospitalizations (179,806), urgent care visitations (136,486), and doctor office visits (207,576). I also listed the number of injuries people sustained. According to VAERS, those injuries are anaphylaxis (10,064), Bell's palsy (16,104), miscarriages (5,078), heart attacks (16,830), myocarditis/pericarditis (52,896), permanently disabled (58,630), thrombocytopenia/low platelet (9,108), life-threatening (34,304), severe allergic reaction (44,999), and shingles (14,830).

---

[13] Ibid.

In this email, I also included the number of California injuries (82,824) and deaths (639), according to States Summaries - OpenVAERS webpage.[14]

I concluded my October 13, 2022, email by sadly noting there were 31,330 deaths.

I also stated the small pox vaccine program for healthcare workers back in 2003 was halted just after two deaths, according to an August 22, 2003, New Scientist article.[15] I noted some medical subject experts indicated VAERS data reflected a small number of actual injuries and deaths.

I told CDPH Assistant Director that Media Team Supervisor responded at 4:14 p.m. on October 20, 2022, to the email I sent to OPA Deputy Director.

In summary, Media Team Supervisor stated my concern "is in conflict with the Department's stance and research findings on vaccination." He embedded a link describing COVID-19 communication policies for CDPH employees for me "to learn more about CDPH's official position." He indicated, "Management team will not have any additional response to your questions." He directed me to "please refrain from sending these types of email communications in the future." He stated he was "concerned your personal research efforts may be a misuse of both state time and equipment."

Now I didn't share this with CDPH Assistant Director on August 24, 2023, but with all due respect to Media Team Supervisor—who I believe was acting reluctantly on

---

[14] Ibid, as of October 3, 2022.

[15] Debora MacKenzie, "US smallpox vaccination plan grinds to a halt," New Scientist, August 22, 2003.

behalf of Deputy Director—his concern: "your personal research efforts may be a misuse of both state time and equipment" veiled threat on October 20, 2022 of filing disciplinary action against me was insulting. I come from good stock.

My mother—before she was my mother—sat in front of a bus more than three years before Rosa Parks! If you recall Parks refused to sit in the colored section on a Mobile, Alabama, bus on December 1, 1955. Dora L. Holmes, who would later become Dora L. Owens after marrying my father Ronald F. Owens, sat in the front of a San Antonio, Texas, city bus twice when she was a twenty-two-year-old WAF (Women in the Air Force).

Whites got on the bus, saw the five-foot-eleven WAF sitting in the front, and scowled at her. She didn't move to the back of the bus, even though the glares and stares of white passengers tried to intimidate her to do so. Just like she wasn't intimidated by white bus passengers, I wasn't going to allow my two managers to intimidate me, especially since I was doing my job.

I noted in that August 24, 2023, email to CDPH Assistant Director that the optics here were quite concerning. A Latino (Becerra) informed two African-American women (Biden Administration Domestic Policy Advisor Susan Rice/Office of Management and Budget Director Shalanda Young) before thousands of viewers on The White House's official YouTube channel that COVID-19 "vaccines are killing people of color . . ." A black man (me) warned two white superiors (Deputy Director and Media Team Supervisor) of this alarming news. One white superior (Media Team Supervisor), acting reluctantly on behest of his white superior (Deputy Director), threatened the black subordinate (me) with disciplinary action because the subordinate (me) informed them of a statement made by a federal governmental health official, publicly commenting about the risks of the COVID-19 vaccine. Secretary Becerra's comments had implications affecting the lives of racial minorities as well as white Americans.

The data I provided was from federal websites documenting COVID-19 vaccine risks. And the question I asked whether the public should be informed of these risks—so they could make decisions for themselves and their children—did not fall under "personal research efforts."

Like I revealed in my ivermectin email months earlier I reiterate that my March 2009 "State of California – Health and Human Services Agency/Department of Health Services Public Information Officer II Duty Statement" states I am to advise "department staff of the public relations implications of department policy decisions."

In addition to being accused of potential wrongdoing, management directing me to "please refrain from sending these types of email communications in the future" directly conflicts with 20 percent of my "essential functions," as stipulated in my "Duty Statement."

Simply put, I was doing my job, yet I was threatened with disciplinary action because of it.

I was transparent with CDPH Assistant Director in that email. I stated during the past few months that I had been emotionally tormented about hearing so many people dying suddenly or unexpectedly.

Furthermore I shared that the mother (Dr. Barbara E. Cahoon-Young) of my sister-in-law (Stephanie Owens) I anonymously referenced in my April 18, 2022, email to OPA Deputy Director was injected with two Moderna COVID-19 vaccines in March 2021. My sister-in-law's mother, Dr. Cahoon-Young, died on July 4, 2021, of severe pulmonary hypertension resulting in congestive heart failure.

Dr. Cahoon-Young was a public health professional. She graduated summa cum laude at the University of California, Berkeley's School of Public Health. She was a public health scientist at the Alameda County Public Health Department. She also studied AIDS at an Oakland clinic and conducted research on Hepatitis C.

The then-Department of Health Services, now the California Department of Public Health, certified Dr. Cahoon-Young on February 8, 2002, to be a public health microbiologist at its Richmond, California, Public Health Laboratory. She retired as Placer County Public Health's Public Health Lab Director on July 14, 2010. It's been more than two years, and my sister-in-law, her husband/ my brother Leonard Owens, and the rest of our family are still grieving Barbara's death, which occurred exactly three weeks after the death of Leonard's and my mother.

That's why I dedicated this book to Dr. Barbara E. Cahoon-Young.

I told CDPH Assistant Director on that 3 p.m., August 22, 2023, Media Team Afternoon Inbox Triage Teams (virtual) meeting that there was a discussion amongst my colleagues about whether VAERS was credible in indicating COVID-19 vaccine injuries and deaths. Feeling the emotional weight of so many people, particularly Dr. Cahoon-Young, who have died or have been injured from COVID-19 vaccines the past couple years, I felt compelled to share with team members what Secretary Becerra said.

I was so emotional that afternoon that I bumbled and messed up Secretary Becerra's quote. And to exacerbate my inarticulateness Deputy Director rudely interrupted and talked over me. She tried to stop me from divulging to my team members what Secretary Becerra said more than sixteen months earlier.

Despite Deputy Director talking over me, I was able to interject that Becerra's comment is still on the White House's official YouTube Channel, which hopefully to my team members legitimized my information and authenticated my concern.

Deputy Director repeatedly asked me to stop talking. She directed Media Team Supervisor to terminate the call. I said I would not stop talking because it was the truth. However, the call was abruptly terminated at about 3:20 p.m. According to my recollection, those who witnessed the incident were five Information Officer 2s, two Information Officer 1s, an Assistant Deputy Director, and an Associate Governmental Program Analyst.

I explained to CDPH Assistant Director that Media Team Supervisor sent me a disciplinary email on August 23, 2023, about my "inappropriate conduct and insubordination," again, probably acting reluctantly on behest of Deputy Director. I also explained to CDPH Assistant Director that Media Team Supervisor falsely accused me of sharing my "personal beliefs about the effectiveness of COVID-19 vaccines." I was told that I was "discussing this misinformation." Moving forward, I was "directed to always remain professional, courteous, and to refrain from making statements which could be perceived as the department's official position."

I noted to CDPH Assistant Director that I failed to understand how relaying comments made by a federal government official constitutes "personal beliefs" and "misinformation." I didn't share my opinion. I shared what Secretary Becerra said, and I backed up what Becerra said with data from federal government websites. I was merely the messenger. My responsibility to my supervisors was to share information they need to know.

I shared with CDPH Assistant Director that Media Team Supervisor showed good leadership by encouraging subordinates (my colleagues and friends) to share information he might not necessarily want to know but needed to know.

In an email he sent to me on August 24, 2023, Media Team Supervisor acknowledged that he shared my concern with Human Resources that I was facing discrimination in the workplace from the Office of Communications management team. He reminded me of my rights. He stated that if I felt I was being discriminated against or subjected to a hostile work environment, I had the right to report a complaint with the Department's Civil Rights Unit.

I told CDPH Assistant Director that it was my duty as a CDPH Information Officer 2 to elevate this issue with her so CDPH senior leadership, California Health and Human Services Agency officials, and the Administration be made aware of Secretary Xavier Becerra's concerning comments, plus supporting VAERS data, and inform them of the false accusations and retaliatory efforts of my management team.

In closing, I noted this sobering data. As of August 11, 2023, more than 1.5 million (precisely 1,585,094) people had been injured, and there had been 35,911 deaths as a result of the COVID-19 vaccine.

These are the concerning thoughts that flooded my mind while I sat in Kaiser that August Friday evening.

I scanned Kaiser's emergency room. I looked at other patients, many of whom were people of color. I thought that they would have liked to have heard from their California Department of Public Health that a Biden Administration official said COVID-19 vaccines were killing people of color at twice the rate of White Americans. But CDPH leadership, who had privy to that information for themselves, denied that same information to Kaiser's emergency room patients, Kaiser hospital staff, and 40 million Californians.

The evening waned. I sat there, waited patiently and thought. It should be easy for public health officials to state that there are COVID-19 vaccine risks, especially for people with pre-existing conditions. If they take the vaccine, it could injure or kill them. Well, lady and gentlemen Readers and Listeners I am one of them. If I took the COVID-19 vaccine, it could possibly paralyze me or probably put me six feet under, which is precisely why I was at Kaiser's emergency room!

It is morally wrong for the powers that be to force people to inject a substance in their bodies that could kill them, and if they don't get injected, they're barred from participating in society. That's a different kind of evil discrimination, and as a Black man, I was, still am, and will always be particularly attuned to it and fight it.

That's why I've doggedly defended truth in these Office of Communications discussions because someone had to speak within the California Department of Public Health (CDPH). Maybe somebody else is speaking up, I don't know. Since we're socially distanced and teleworking, I just don't know. I would like to think there are other

CDPH employees who, just like me, have represented the interests of forty million Californians by countering lies and speaking truth for them.

Finally a nurse walked up to me and beckoned me to come with her. This was an encouraging sign because more than four years earlier, it was the doctor who walked up to me, told me to follow him to his office, and sit down in the wheelchair waiting for me. He directed the nurse to wheel me in the emergency room because tests indicated that I had blood clots in both of my lungs, and I needed immediate treatment.

That was not the case on that August 25, 2023, cool summer evening. The emergency room doctor determined that there weren't any blood clots as there had been on February 23, 2019. My leg still hurt. But thank the LORD, at least there weren't any blood clots. I guess my physical condition was a result of the intense emotional stress I experienced that week.

I called my dad, told him the good news, apprised other family members and notified friends. That next day I awoke, got up and walked 4.4 miles between 10 a.m. and noon at the park pedestrian track near the house. I slowly walked more than eight laps around that hardpan track. I held my iPhone in my right hand, spoke into the microphone, and recorded one hour and twenty-eight minutes of monologue in a transcription app. That physically energetic exercise period and emotionally cathartic recording session laid the foundation of *Muzzled Truth*.

Days transpired. I did not think that I would ever receive a response from my email. But, surprisingly, I did on September 6, 2023.

It was she, California Department of Public Health's Assistant Director, who thanked me for reaching out and sharing my concerns.

CDPH Assistant Director offered condolences on the loss of my family member, stated that I had the right to file a complaint if I felt I was being discriminated against or harassed, and included a list of CDPH Employee Complaint Resources on the Department's intranet.

CDPH Assistant Director also indicated I may also utilize the services provided by the Employee Assistance Program for any needed support.

In response to the information I provided related to COVID-19 vaccines, CDPH Assistant Director also stated, "The department relies on scientific and medical experts when formulating public health guidance and policies."

CDPH Assistant Director added that these experts rely on data and provide information on all aspects of medical interventions.

"The Office of Communications team is not positioned to be able to advise on the technical, scientific aspects of COVID-19 vaccines," CDPH Assistant Director wrote in her September 6, 2023, email response. "It is appropriate for management to direct the team to focus on their role."

In an afterthought comment intended to downplay the urgency of the concern I conveyed, CDPH Assistant Director stated as an "FYI -I did view the video you referenced. '_It appears_' [italics/underline added] that Secretary Becerra misspoke and was actually discussing deaths associated with COVID-19, not the vaccines."

She thanked me "for sharing your concerns." She encouraged me "to work with your management team to clarify your role and responsibility within the Office of Communications."

With her writing, "*it appears,*" CDPH Assistant Director gaslighted me.

Essentially, CDPH Assistant Director said I didn't actually hear what Becerra said. For a split second, I even questioned my own sanity. Did I hear what I heard? Then it hit me. "Wait a minute! I won't let them do this to me. I did hear what I heard and Becerra said what he said! Besides, what about all those thousands of COVID-19 vaccine injuries and those thousands of COVID-19 vaccine deaths indicated on VAERS?" CDPH Assistant Director ignored VAERS.

Let's just say, for the sake of discussion, that Health and Human Services Secretary Becerra misspoke. How come he didn't stumble or stutter or correct himself?

Remember the two African-American women (Biden Administration Domestic Policy Advisor Susan Rice/ Office of Management and Budget Director Shalanda Young) who sat there listening to Becerra? They did not react. They did not ask or say he misspoke. They did not inquire whether he made a mistake. They did not request clarification. No one said anything, yet someone, anyone, everyone should have said something!

And again, let's just say, for the sake of discussion, that the Health and Human Services Secretary misspoke. I repeat: what... about...VAERS?

Quite frankly, I think it's disrespectful to thousands of COVID-19-vaccinated injured and thousands of COVID-19-vaccinated dead. VAERS gave them voice, and CDPH Assistant Director completely ignored and essentially muzzled them.

Essentially, CDPH Assistant Director *Muzzled Truth*!

But since the culture of CDPH has been to ignore mama bears and papa bears and their vaccine-injured and dead children, how else did I think COVID-19 vaccine victims were going to be treated? COVID-19-injured and COVID-19-dead people are an impediment for CDPH executing its COVID-19 vaccine agenda.

Quite frankly, it was insulting to be told I did not hear what I heard. But it's not about the messenger. It's about the message.

What is particularly irksome is three people—CDPH Assistant Director, Office of Communications Deputy Director and Media Team Supervisor—had privy to potentially lifesaving information that was denied to 40 million Californians, particularly Californians of color.

I am disgusted! (Deep exhale.)

It was I, Ronald Owens, who was vexed, saddened, outraged, depressed, and, yes, disgusted that California Department of Public Health leadership knew that COVID-19 vaccines were killing people but neglected to do anything about it.

CHAPTER 8
Counseling Memorandum

It was he, Office of Communications Media Team Supervisor, who informed me in a one-on-one virtual meeting that I would be emailed a Counseling Memorandum because of what I said on August 22, 2023.

On September 22, 2023, at 11:30 a.m., Media Team Supervisor said he wanted to give me a heads up that I would be issued a Counseling Memorandum. During our conversation—held virtually on our respective state-issued laptop computers—we talked about my COVID-19 vaccine concerns.

Minutes after we concluded our approximate thirty-minute meeting, Media Team Supervisor emailed me the Counseling Memorandum. I saw that the incoming email arrived at 12:07 p.m. I deeply exhaled and opened the email. That one-page document, dated the day before on September 21, 2023, was officially addressed to Information Officer II Ron Owens. The document was from Media Team Supervisor.

I paused and reflected on our recent conversation. I also reflected on previous conversations. While I appreciate Media Team Supervisor talking to me before emailing me the Counseling Memorandum, and while I understand as well as empathize that he probably acted on behest of Deputy Director, if I was in his position, I would have stood up for subordinate and not have signed the document.

Even though he disagreed with me, Media Team Supervisor repeatedly told me that he had no problems with me sharing my COVID-19 vaccine concerns. I appreciate audible words, but silent actions would have spoken much louder.

The fact that he signed Counseling Memorandum causes me to wonder whether he truly had no problems listening to my warnings about COVID-19 vaccines. His name was on the Counseling Memorandum. Did he exclusively write it, or did Office of Communications Deputy Director or Assistant Deputy Director (or perhaps an attorney) write it, as I suspected?

I started to read it. The Counseling Memorandum discussed "your insubordinate and discourteous conduct." Essentially I was being counseled, censured, and corrected for informing my Information Officer colleagues in last month's meeting that the Department of Health and Human Services Secretary Xavier Becerra said we know these vaccines are killing people of color . . . at about two times the rate of White Americans.

"This memo is further intended to direct you in immediately correcting this concern," the document, printed on official CDPH letterhead, didactically declared.

I paused and reflected again. Exactly a month earlier (August 22, 2023), I shared with team members— seven Information Officers, an Associate Governmental Program Analyst, the Assistant Deputy Director, Media

Team Supervisor, plus Deputy Director—what was on my heart during our daily meeting.

My heart was sad about Dr. Barbara Cahoon-Young, who was my sister-in-law's (Stephanie Owens) mother. Dr. Cahoon-Young died on July 4, 2021, of severe pulmonary hypertension resulting in congestive heart failure. While we don't absolutely, positively, incontrovertibly, and indubitably know her death was associated with her taking COVID-19 vaccines, her death occurred more than four months after receiving two Moderna COVID-19 vaccines.

So, on August 22, 2023, team members discussed a *California Globe* media inquiry at that 3 p.m. Media Team Afternoon Inbox Triage Teams (virtual) meeting. During that discussion, they questioned whether VAERS is credible indicating COVID-19 vaccine injuries and deaths. I don't understand why VAERS—Vaccine Adverse Events Reporting System—is not considered credible because it is co-managed by the Centers for Disease Control and Prevention.

I remember feeling frustrated about the discussion because the tonality of the meeting seemed to be dismissive of those who filed VAERS reports. I also remember feeling the emotional weight of knowing about so many people who died suddenly or died unexpectedly the past couple of years. I just couldn't take it anymore. The heated feelings of anger, sadness, exasperation, and nervousness welled within me and, like volcanic lava, erupted out of me. So I shared what Secretary Becerra said. However, Office of Communications management rejected the message and rudely repudiated me, the messenger.

Back to Thursday, September 22, 2023—I continued to read the email the Media Team Supervisor had just sent me.

"This documentation sets forth measures for addressing these issues in an effort to resolve them," the document asserted. "This Counseling Memorandum is not intended to be disciplinary in nature."

The Counseling Memorandum cited three examples to buttress the assertion that I exhibited "insubordinate and discourteous conduct."

I expressed my "personal views that perhaps there was truth to information that is contrary to the department's stance" during the August 1 team meeting. I stated twice "that 'all politicians lie' or words to that effect" during the August 17 team meeting. And I shared "personal beliefs about the effectiveness of COVID-19 vaccines in response to a media inquiry" during the August 22 team meeting.

The Counseling Memorandum repeatedly stated that I was sharing "personal beliefs," and the document reminded me that I'm "not to share personal beliefs" and was to stop "sharing misinformation about the vaccine in the workplace."

These Counseling Memorandum statements are all outright lies!

I shared what a presidential cabinet official said. I cited data from a federal website. How is that my personal belief?

If the California Department of Public Health's Office of Communications management lies to the most tenured, the most experienced, and at more than sixty-six years old, probably the eldest Office of Communications staff member, what other lies have been told and are being told to 40 million Californians?

"You are again directed to separate your personal beliefs, including but not limited to those related to the COVID-19 vaccination, from your job duties at CDPH as an Information Officer II," the Counseling Memorandum stated. "The department relies on scientific and medical experts when formulating public health guidance and policies. The study and analysis of vaccine effectiveness, and the formulation of public health guidance is not within the scope of an Information Officer II.'"

Question: But if millions of people are being injured and thousands of people are dying from COVID-19 vaccines, shouldn't the information of CDPH's scientific and medical experts be questioned by CDPH's critical thinking Information Officers who could field reporter questions on this topic?

The Counseling Memorandum stated that I am "to speak in a matter that is respectful and professional to your colleagues and chain-of-command." I am "to follow the direction provided, including the direction to not share personal beliefs at team meetings."

Even though I am sixty-six years old, and although I have worked for CDPH for more than fourteen years, I felt like I was being talked to like a child. I resented the fact that they were making it about lone me anyway. The issue is not about me. The issue is about the millions of people who are suffering from COVID-19 vaccines, which California Department of Public Health officials and news releases and CDPH ads repeatedly declare "is safe and effective."

The Counseling Memorandum stated that my "conduct during the team meeting was unacceptable and will not be tolerated by the Department."

The Counseling Memorandum concluded that this "is not intended to constitute adverse action. However, the Department may take adverse action against you for the incidents cited in this memo, as well as any future incidents."

The Counseling Memorandum was to be placed in my Official Personnel File for a period of one year. After a year, I may request that it be removed with management approval. I was asked to "please sign below to indicate that you have received a copy of this memo, and that I have met with you to discuss its contents."

The repeated mantra that I keep expressing "my personal beliefs" is patently false, and I'll repeat, it is a lie!

According to the Counseling Memorandum, I was insubordinate. However, the Counseling Memorandum did not specify how I was insubordinate, according to federal law, state statute, or departmental policy.

If I was insubordinate, I wouldn't have gone up my chain of command. I would have sent my COVID-19-vaccine-is-not-safe-and-effective emails to the Center for Infectious Diseases Deputy Director, who is California's State Epidemiologist. If I was insubordinate, I would have emailed my emails to CDPH Senior Leadership (the Directorate), all Deputy Directors and Assistant Deputy Directors, something that I do everyday when I email the Office of Communications Daily Media Updates. And if I was insubordinate I would have emailed all CDPH employees. Despite the emergency of the situation, I alerted superiors through my chain of command.

According to the Counseling Memorandum, I was discourteous. But it was Deputy Director who created a hostile work environment and was discourteous to me. During the August 22, 2023, meeting, Deputy Director tried to prevent me from talking, repeatedly interrupted me while I was talking, and was successful in directing Media Team Supervisor to shut down the call while I was speaking in mid-sentence.

According to the Counseling Memorandum, I offered my personal views to what Comms Deputy Director said about conspiracy theories. I do not specifically recall what I said, but I do remember saying that "all politicians lie."

I made that statement in the context of responding to another Information Officer 2, who remarked about a headline that reported President Donald Trump had been indicted. Information Officer 2 offered his personal opinion about that particular news story that castigated President Trump. Concerned about the incessant political and legal persecution of President Trump I casually remarked that politicians—I was actually thinking about Joe Biden, Gavin Newsom, Congress and State Legislature—on both sides of the political aisle lie. I'm not breaking any news here, folks! Millions of Americans say politicians lie every day.

Throughout my almost thirty-year state service career, I kept silent while coworkers on the ideological left opined on politics in the workplace. I bit my tongue. I remained silent while they criticized, for example, Republicans. I bit my tongue. One coworker incessantly mocked Alaska Gov. Sarah Palin after she lost her vice presidential bid. I bit my tongue. I'm at the sunset of a nearly thirty-year state service career and less than six months away from commemorating my fifteen-year anniversary at CDPH, and quite frankly, I just got sick and tired of biting swollen tongue! So I merely said all politicians lie.

Information Officer 2 also offered his personal opinion at a June 23, 2022, 9:45 a.m. staff meeting as well. I am unable to quote him verbatim, but it had to do with him offering condolences to coworkers who felt sad about the Supreme Court's ruling on abortion. I would have liked to have offered another perspective during that meeting. I would have liked to have said that family planning and abortion is a racist policy.

In a one-on-one conversation later on June 23, 2022, I told Media Team Supervisor about the inappropriateness of Information Officer 2's comments. I explained that there's another side to the abortion issue. I said family planning—and, eventually, abortion—was introduced in the United States to curtail the birth of the descendants of slaves. I shared with Media Team Supervisor about MAAFA 21, a 2009 documentary that reports the 150 years of black genocidal history.[16]

I asked Media Team Supervisor if I could send him information so he could view MAAFA 21. He declined. However, Media Team Supervisor said during that June 23, 2022 conversation, that he appreciated me not offering my personal opinion.

Back to reading the Counseling Memorandum on September 22, 2023—so, Information Officer 2 (who is white) is allowed to express his personal opinion, yet I (who is black) am censored and punished for offering mine?How is that fair? CDPH constantly emphasizes racial and cultural diversity, equity, and inclusion, but

---

[16] Crutcher, Mark, director. "MAAFA 21: Black Genocide in 21st Century America" documentary.

the department—indeed all of California state civil service— needs to also place emphasis on ideological diversity, equity, and inclusion.

According to the Counseling Memorandum, I have been discussing and sharing "your personal beliefs" about COVID-19 vaccines. CDPH management are calling the facts I have raised to be my "personal beliefs." Again, I ask, how does the Department of Health and Human Services Secretary Xavier Becerra's video-recorded statement (which is still on the White House's official YouTube channel for all to see and hear): "we know these vaccines are killing people . . ." constitues "personal beliefs?" How is sharing data from a federal website, co-managed by the Center for Disease Control and Prevention, my "personal beliefs?" These are facts. I raised them.

It is actually "personal belief" to repeatedly say, "COVID-19 vaccines are safe and effective," when, clearly, according to Becerra, VAERS data, censured news reports, social media posts, and anecdotal[17] accounts about people being injured and dying suddenly, they are not.

It is unfortunate that the Office of Comms top management has made the issue about the messenger and not the more important injury-sparing and life-saving message.

"Withhold not good from them to whom it is due, when it is in the power of thine hand to do it," states Proverbs 3:27, which as I previously noted is one of my man codes.

It is morally reprehensible that the Office of Comms top management has withhold, is withholding, and to this date is continuing to withhold from 40 million Californians about them learning that millions of people

---

[17] Sharp, Jennifer, director. "ANECDOTALS" documentary.

have been injured and thousands of people have died from COVID-19 vaccines.

I am disgusted! (Deep exhale.)

While writing this section of *Muzzled Truth* I learned officials at the White House, the Centers for Disease Control and Prevention (CDC), the American Academy of Pediatricians and others knew way back in May 2021 that COVID-19 vaccines were injuring and killing people![18]

But they—particularly Dr. Anthony Fauci and CDC Director Dr. Rochelle Walensky—lied and continued to declare "vaccines are safe and effective!"

Now we know why Secretary Becerra said what he said nearly a year later (April 14, 2022). Becerra knew!

So no, CDPH Assistant Director, Becerra did not misspeak!

Public Information Officers (PIOs), particularly those employed at the California Department of Public Health, need to challenge official narratives, be critical thinkers, be courageous challengers and speak up.

And senior department leaders who manage their PIOs need to create a climate whereby PIOs hold frank discussions and not be afraid "from making statements which could be perceived as the department's official position," such as what the Office of Communications management emailed me. That managerial mindset is not conducive in fostering a healthy workplace environment.

---

[18] Amy Kelly, "FOIA'd Emails Reveal Highest-Level Leaders at White House, HHS, CDC, NIAID, AAP All Knew COVID Vaccines Linked to Myocarditis, Yet Publicly Covered Up Findings," DailyClout, October 18, 2023.

That managerial mindset chills our U.S. Constitution First Amendment right to freedom of speech.

Perhaps Deputy Directors (DD) and Assistant Deputy Directors (ADD)—particularly those law enforcement, first responder, emergency services and public health government agencies—should not be political appointees. Perhaps DDs and ADDs should be held by state employees who hold civil service classifications. So, then DDs and ADDs would not be beholden to the shifting political agenda of the governors who appoint them.

During this saga, I once mentioned to Media Team Supervisor that we're PIOs—Public Information Officers. We're not PIOs—Propagandist Information Officers.

It is I, Public Information Officer Ron Owens, who begrudgingly acknowledged receipt of this Counseling Memorandum, emphatically disagreed with it, declined to sign it, and, yes, am disgusted about it.

Signing this document would be admitting that I had been offering "personal beliefs" and acknowledging that "COVID-19 vaccines are safe and effective," which is a lie!

CHAPTER 9

Germans Like Us Implemented "The Final Solution"

When I last visited Yad Vashem (Holocaust Memorial Museum) in Jerusalem, Israel, in the summer of 2008, I learned that the Germans who implemented "The Final Solution to the Jewish Question" weren't just the brown-shirted Nazi Party storm troopers, nor the grayish, green-uniformed German soldiers, nor the black clad/trimmed in white SS.

The German Nazis who implemented "The Final Solution"—or looked the other way while six million Jews plus six million others were exterminated—were Catholic or Protestant middle-class, college-educated, law-abiding, and tax-paying people like you and me.

Recalling my third visit to Yad Vashem—I first visited the Holocaust Memorial Museum in 1996 and then in 2000—I've reflected on the past three years.

If I had the supernatural ability to place the people I've encountered from 2020 to 2023 into Nazi Germany during World War II, the people who implemented the Holocaust could have been:

- COVID cops employed at Costco, Sam's Club, Target, or Walmart

- Downtown Sacramento mail and shipping employee who ejected me from his business for not wearing a face mask

- Local grocery store woman who told me to wear a mask because door signage ordered customers to do so

- A See's Candies sales associate who told my late eighty-nine-year-old multiple myeloma-battling mother pushing a walker to raise her face mask to cover her nose, which smothered her inhaling and exhaling and caused her to hyperventilate

- H&R Block receptionist who cited Centers for Disease Control and Prevention guidelines when she told me to remove my impenetrable plastic shield and put on a pervious paper face mask

- Elk Grove Subway Sandwich maker who argued with me, berated me, and ejected me from his store into the frigid night for not wearing a face mask

- Two Lowe's shoppers who stared at me, scowled at me, and said something between themselves about me being unmasked while I walked by them

- White female anti-police protestor at Sacramento's Capitol Park who offered me a face mask, and I reflectively retorted, "Like George Floyd, I need to breathe!"

- Workers who shouted and shamed those of us who refused to wear face masks

- Pastors who capitulated to the government and closed down their churches

- Clergy who coerced congregates to get the COVID-19 vaccine as an act of love because Jesus Christ would have done so, even though according to their own Bible, Jesus healed countless people from their diseases

- Citizens who proudly declared they received the jab and castigated those of us who didn't get the jab, and after they got the jab and boosters, they contracted COVID-19 anyway

- Employers who forced their employees to get the COVID-19 vaccines, or they would be terminated

- Employees who wore masks and got tested and received jabs and got boosted to keep their jobs

- People who started off strong in their resolve and resisted government masking, social distancing, testing, and jabbing mandates yet weakened anyway

- DMV security guard (note Chapter 10) who shouted at me to remove my impermeable motorcycle helmet from my entire head and strap on a flimsy paper face mask just to cover my nose and mouth.

- California Department of Public Health management who ignored me, threatened disciplinary action against me, and muzzled me for telling them that on April 14, 2022, Department of Health and Human Services Secretary Becerra said: "We know that [COVID-19] vaccines are killing people of color, Black, Latinos, Indigenous People at about two times the rate of White Americans!"

Now we know how so many German citizens sat idly by and either allowed or participated in the extermination of more than 12 million people. Now we need not ask, with self-righteous verbal tone, how could they have committed genocide?

CHAPTER 10
Face Mask Argument

It was he, a Department of Motor Vehicles field office security guard, who loudly commanded me to remove my thick motorcycle helmet and put on a thin blue paper face mask.

On February 14, 2022, I rode my 2021 Can-Am Spyder, a two tires in front and one tire in rear touring motorcycle, to pick up my personalized California Legacy plates at Sacramento DMV Field Office on Broadway. I had ordered the black and gold plates online nine months earlier. There was a backlog because of the pandemic, so I was really excited to finally affix an alphanumeric truncated license plate character combination denoting my Sea-to-Sky at the back of my unit.

It was an overcast cool, yet not terribly uncomfortable Monday afternoon ride. I was slightly concerned that I might encounter someone who would insist that I wear a face mask. But I was confident that I would be left alone—if I only kept my black matte Schuberth C3 Pro helmet strapped on my head and kept my face shield lowered.

This was not the first time I wore my motorcycle helmet when I entered establishments that mandated customers wear face masks. I was not opposed to continue making a stand and not comply to face mask mandates, as I had done many times before. But as we motorcycle riders know, sometimes it's just convenient to keep the helmet on our heads when, for example, darting in and out of a convenience mart or grocery store.

I draped the travel cover over my Spyder, deeply exhaled, and walked across the parking lot to the DMV field office front door entrance. There was a serpentine line of people standing and quietly waiting. They were standing there muted, all wearing blue face masks. I stood there for a few moments, hoping I would blend in and not be noticed.

"You need to put on a face mask," Security Guard loudly commanded me.

I couldn't believe it. I remember thinking: "He actually wants me to remove my motorcycle helmet to put on a face mask?"

A heated conversation immediately ensued. I repeatedly asked him with my face shield lowered, "What is better: wearing a motorcycle helmet or putting on a paper face mask?" He didn't answer the question. Security Guard pulled his smartphone out of his pocket and showed me his screen, which displayed DMV's mask-wearing policy.

I tried to reason with Security Guard. A few moments of more intense discussion ensued, which was witnessed by about twenty other mask-wearing DMV customers. Even though I was angry at him for berating me, I still kept my cool while I tried to reason with him.

One of my man codes is not to view negative interactions with white people within the context of race. But I have to be honest with you. A quasi-law enforcement white man berating me triggered instances of police berating black men. Now I realize this wasn't about race from Security Guard's perspective. But from my perspective, the incident trigged unpleasant childhood memories, when white people viewed me by the color of my skin rather than judge me by the content of my character.

After Security Guard saw that I was not going to comply, he left. He came back moments later holding a blue face mask. He extended his hand and wanted me to take it. But I did not reach for it.

First of all, judging by his overweight condition and noticing perspiration droplets percolating on his forehead and face, I didn't think he was healthy nor hygienic for me to accept him handing me a face mask that was going to be pressed on my lips. I made this immediate observation while at the same time feeling sorry for him for having to wear a face mask.

Secondly, I was not going to make it difficult for me to breathe. I had blood clots in both of my lungs more than three years earlier, and I simply was not going to imperil my health.

Security Guard disappeared again. My anxiety level increased just a little because I momentarily thought he was going after a Sacramento City police officer or Sacramento County Sheriff's deputy. What was I going to do if real law enforcement came on the scene, I thought. I wanted to still stand my ground, but would I have the courage to do so?

Fortunately, that question was never answered. He went to management instead because DMV Manager eventually came out with another blue paper face mask in her hand. DMV Manager asked me to put it on. I respectfully declined. I showed her a screenshot of my face mask medical exemption that was archived in the camera roll of my iPhone.

"Ron is under my care and has a medical condition that precludes him from wearing a mask or a face shield," a physician wrote for me the previous year. "He is exempt under the California UNRUH act as well as the ADA from wearing a face covering of any kind. HIPAA privacy laws protect him from having to reveal the details of his health condition."

I will not divulge the identity of the physician who, after examining me, issued me that face mask medical exemption.

As you know, I have already revealed that I was diagnosed with deep vein thrombosis, and in February 2019, tests indicated that I had blood clots in both of my lungs.

DMV Manager backed off. She said I may have to wait outside until all the customers left the field office after DMV Employee screened me.

"Fine," I said.

I stood in line with my motorcycle helmet still on and face shield still lowered. When I reached DMV Employee who screens incoming customers, she also asked me to wear a blue face mask. I politely declined. I told her I have a medical exemption and proceeded to show her. She glanced at it and didn't contest me any further. She processed me in and assigned me a public counter appointment number.

Seeking to avoid any further confrontation, I immediately exited the front door of the DMV field office and sat on the bench outside. I actually felt slightly lightheaded and out of breath. I noticed my heart pulse rate had increased. Motorcycle helmets aren't designed for occupants to talk loudly in a heated argument. As we riders can certainly attest, motorcycle helmets are specifically designed for occupants to just sit, relax, and quietly enjoy the ride. Since I was outside, I lifted my face shield to physically recover from arguing with Security Guard. I also needed to calm down and cool down.

A few moments transpired. Security Guard 2 approached me. Apparently, she witnessed the heated verbal exchange between Security Guard and me. Security Guard 2 apologized for Security Guard berating me. Security Guard 2 agreed with me and my helmet-wearing position. I thanked Security Guard 2. We introduced ourselves and shook hands.

I went inside DMV at 4:57 p.m., three minutes before they closed and locked the doors. I sat inside the field office wearing my plastic, fiberglass, Kevlar, and carbon fiber motorcycle helmet. I had lowered my polycarbonate face shield before entering the front door. I discreetly raised it a little to get some air. Not wanting to encounter Security Guard again or deal with any other DMV COVID cop, I lowered face shield and sat patiently—waiting for my number to be called.

I saw one Russian-speaking DMV customer with her paper face mask understandably positioned below her nose so she could breathe. My heart went out to her. She eventually pulled it off with exasperation as I heard her speak in Russian to her companion.

Yet Security Guard, who demanded a few minutes earlier that I remove my hermetically sealed motorcycle helmet and strap on a razor-thin paper face mask, was nowhere to be found. Good for Russian woman. Good for me. Good for all of us DMV customers. Let there be peace in the valley!

I sat there and thought about this absurd and illogical face mask-wearing policy. "Are they trying to kill us by suffocating us all to death?" I rhetorically asked myself. If the purpose of a face mask is to protect people from COVID-19 aerosolized pathogens diffused in that DMV waiting room, a person wearing a $700 motorcycle helmet with a lowered face shield that is the same material as fighter jet canopies is a lot more protective than a person wearing a paper twenty-five-cent face mask!

It was I, a motorcycle rider, who refused to comply to a DMV field office security guard's command to remove my thick motorcycle helmet to put on a thin blue paper face mask.

AFTERWORD

It is imperative to review what federal, state, and local government officials did to us during the COVID-19 pandemic so we will never forget.

They told us to stay home. They restricted our movements. They took away livelihoods. They destroyed small Mom-and-Pop stores. They corralled us to shop at Target, Walmart, Sam's Club, and Costco Big-box stores. They took away jobs. They crashed booming economy.

They denied some to visit their elders in skilled nursing facilities. They allowed some seniors to die alone there. They even prevented funerals and exacerbated the grief-stricken from grieving and burying their loved ones.

They disrupted families. They separated schoolmates and wedged playmates. They ostracized girls and boys from interacting, fostering relationships and blossoming friendships with other boys and girls.

They stopped little league baseball and soccer leagues. They cancelled track meets, baseball games and other organized sports at K-12 schools, community colleges and universities. They prevented fans from spectating sports activities at stadiums, arenas and basketball courts. They shut down K-12 schools, community college and university graduations.

They trampled on our constitutional rights. They said we couldn't buy or sell or conduct other commerce. They prevented petitioning. They inhibited politicking. They chided American citizens for peacefully protesting and castigated them for demonstrating to reopen.

They unilaterally changed scores of laws without being introduced/sponsored by legislator(s); without being reviewed by legislative counsel; without studying fiscal impact; without being heard in committee(s); without legislators hearing and analyzing arguments for; without lawmakers listening to and pondering arguments against; without considering opinions of subject matter experts (SMEs) on both sides of the issue; without allowing proponents, opponents and SMEs to introduce oral testimony, written testimony and letters in the public record; without being moved by vote from lower house; without being passed by vote in upper house; and without being signed by the head of the executive branch.

They shut down places of worship. They later dictated to us how we are to worship. They said singing and chanting in church was prohibited.

They required the wearing of cloth, paper like or plastic material face coverings. As a result of these face coverings we didn't see the faces of family members, our own children, passerby's and strangers in public. Passerby's and strangers in public no longer saw the faces of family members and our own children.

People wore face masks outside. Runners wore face masks. Cyclists wore face masks. Even baseball, basketball, football and other professional athletes and referees who officiated them—plus spectators who watched them—all wore face masks. In my common-sense layperson's opinion it's unwise for anyone to wear a face mask while playing sports or exercising.

Face masks divided people and consigned them into two opposing camps. Whether to wear a face mask or not wear a face mask pitted one camp against the other. That caused tension between us and amongst us. That caused each of us to view one another with defensiveness, ire and suspicion. When strangers initially interact with one another, they usually say "Hello, how are you doing?" But during the COVID-19 pandemic arguments ensued upon initial meeting. It was common for people to attack one another for not wearing a face mask.

Masks caused communication problems. We had difficulty hearing and problems understanding words uttered from masked mouths. Masks mask lips. Masks mask smiles. Masks mute voices.

The public health policy of masking should cause us to question. What about masks suppressing inhalation? What about masks restricting exhalation? What about masks causing lightness of head and forgetfulness of thought? Do we know the myriad of other ailments, sickness and diseases that may have developed amongst those who continually wore masks for a prolonged period of time?

The public health policy of social distancing should cause us to question. What about exacerbated human interaction? What about the psychological and physical effects of seniors and the shut-in and singles being incarcerated alone in their houses, apartments, and rooms? What about people being alienated from family and away from friends, coworkers, and people?

Federal, state, and local government officials rewarded face mask wearers and social distance compliers and punished non-face mask wearers and social distance non-compliers. Governmental mandates created the civilian deputization of COVID cops who were stationed at the front doors of corporate box and grocery stores. They encouraged sneering, spying and snitching.

And then to exacerbate matters for these federal, state, and local government officials who mandated that we wear face masks and directed that we socially distance ourselves, California Gov. Gavin Newsom got together with his friends at an expensive restaurant during the COVID-19 pandemic. We saw the color photographs. There he was and his buddies, all sitting closely around a table not wearing face masks and not socially distancing themselves. The optics were very problematic—hypocritical is more of an accurate word.

That Newsom restaurant incident, and a second incident showing the same maskless governor attending a professional football game, demonstrated that masking mandates and social distancing directives were unnecessary.

"A lie doesn't become truth, wrong doesn't become right, and evil doesn't become good, just because it's accepted by a majority," said Booker T. Washington (1856–1915), an American educator, author, orator, and adviser to several US presidents.[19]

South African attorney Dexter Ryneveldt cited this provocative Washington quote on February 5, 2022, during his opening statement at an international Grand Jury that adjudicated COVID-19 crimes committed against

---

[19] Booker T. Washington, Wikipedia, last edited on October 31, 2023.

humanity.[20] The Grand Jury consisted of lawyers, doctors, medical subject matter experts, witnesses, and victims.

According to my layperson understanding, this Grand Jury is similar to a moot or mock court, meaning the evidence presented in thirty-five hours and five minutes of testimony could be presented in an actual court of law or international tribunal.

"What we're undertaking is to give you a complete picture—a complete picture of what has happened and what is happening," said German attorney-at-law Dr. Reiner Fuellmich, of the exhaustive eight-day Grand Jury proceedings. "Because only by seeing the complete picture will you come to the conclusion that we cannot trust those who many of us are used to trusting —our government."[21]

Masking mandates and social distancing directives plus other COVID-19 treatment protocols were lies told as truth and wrong told as right and evil told as good.

It is my Hope that every public health professional who believed and participated in the implementation of social distancing, masking, testing and COVID-19 vaccine rollout would have the intellectual courage and view Grand Jury: The Court of Public Opinion testimony.[22]

Here's the Grand Jury's itinerary:

- February 5, 2022, Day 1: Opening Statements, 1:25:35

---

[20] Google Grand Jury The Court of Public Opinion, Berlin Corona Investigative Committee.

[21] Ibid.

[22] Ibid.

- February 12, 2022, Day 2: Historical Background, 5:47:18

- February 13, 2022, Day 3: PCR-Test, 5:00:57

- February 19, 2022, Day 4: Injections, 5:50:55

- February 20, 2022, Day 5: Financial Destruction, 4:24:06

- February 26, 2022, Day 6: Eugenics & Outlook, 4:22:51

- May 19, 2022, Day 7: Psychology & Propaganda, 4:17:20

- June 9, 2022, Day 8: Closing Arguments, 3:28:03

As time proceeds the general public will have questions and demand answers about what happened, especially since according to the latest Rasmussen Reports twenty-four percent of American adults say they know someone personally who died from side effects of the COVID-19 vaccine.[23]

According to his own research Dr. James Thorp, an obstetrician-gynecologist and maternal fetal medicine specialist who was fired by SSM Health St. Mary's Hospital for telling his pregnant women patients about the dangers of COVID-19 vaccines, estimates between one to five percent of American citizens have been severely injured or killed by COVID-19 vaccines.[24]

---

[23] Rasmussen Reports, "Killer Jab? 24% Say Someone They Know Died From COVID-19 Vaccine," November 2, 2023.

[24] "Pfizer & THE COVENANT WITH DEATH —DR. JAMES THORP," by SGT Report, November 8, 2023 podcast audio.

I applaud Dr. Fuellmich for spearheading and moderating this Grand Jury. All those lawyers, doctors, medical subject matter experts, witnesses, and victims who worked with him answer a lot of questions and raise even more.

I also applaud ANECDOTALS Director Jennifer Sharp. Her 2023 moving human interest documentary is about "a compassionate exploration of the nuanced vaccine debate. While the vaccine debate grows more divided, those with adverse reactions get stuck in the middle."[25]

Sharp, who is COVID-19 vaccine injured, synopsized ANECDOTALS on her website.

> *"In March 2021, after receiving my Pfizer shot, I couldn't feel the left side of my face for a month. Eighteen months later, electric shocks and muscle weakness continue. Unable to receive the 2nd dose, I am amongst a group of partially-vaccinated people who have been outcast from many aspects of society with no empathy. We've been censored and told it's unethical to talk about our stories because we are just anecdotes.*

> *"This movie provides a glimpse into the lives of the Anecdotals—those of us whose lives have been changed drastically by taking the vaccine. It also reflects on the division and politics that prevents us from getting much needed care. Anecdotals is a personal journey that focuses on questions, not answers, and people, not politics."*

---

[25] Google "ANECDOTALS" documentary.

It is also my sincere hope that every *Muzzled Truth* reader and listener—as well as every public health professional— would have the emotional courage to watch ANECDOTALS.

"It's easier to fool people than to convince them that they have been fooled," a quote, commonly attributed to American author Mark Twain, states.[26] I am convinced beyond a shadow of doubt! Viewing the Grand Jury proceedings and watching ANECDOTALS will convince those who were fooled by the COVID-19 official narrative.

It is most unfortunate that Californians were fooled and a lie was accepted as truth by a majority.

We have all been blessed by people before us who stood up against evil and tried to make the world a better place. Well, this was my turn to bless you and bless others. This was my time to stand up. This was my opportunity and try to make the world a better place. I fought for forty million Californians right to know the truth about information that was denied them.

That is why, as Peter A. Baldridge wrote in his Foreword, I spoke "out and acted on behalf of the public that the public health profession ostensibly serves."

Thank you for unmuzzling truth by reading or listening to *Muzzled Truth*!

Ronald F. Owens Jr.
November 13, 2023

---

[26] Did Mark Twain Say 'It's Easier to Fool People Than to Convince Them That They Have Been Fooled'?, Snopes, last modified on December 29, 2016.

ABOUT THE AUTHOR

My first writing job in 1984 was working as Stringer Reporter with *The Grapevine Independent*, Rancho Cordova's general circulation newspaper. I reported on community events, fire protection district, park district, school board district, and wrote feature stories for this local weekly publication.

During the same period, I secured a student assistant position as Editor of *The Pipeline*, an employee newsletter at California State University, Sacramento's (CSUS) Plant Operations Department. I reported on facilities management news and wrote feature stories about employees and the projects they worked on to maintain CSUS. I was pursuing a Bachelor of Arts Degree in Government/Journalism at CSUS at that time.

My first big job after graduating from CSUS in 1986 was as Publications Editor at the California Newspaper Publishers Association (CNPA). I worked at CNPA from 1987 to 1992. Desktop publishing was first introduced in the workplace then, so I learned to produce *California Publisher*, CNPA's trade association monthly publication, on a Macintosh SE computer using PageMaker desktop publishing software. Essentially, I reported on newspaper industry news. The people who owned, managed, provided editorial content, placed ads, produced, sold, and distributed California's newspapers were my exclusive and influential yet very critical readership.

Before each edition, I scripted—with No. 2 pencil—the topic of articles and placement of stories and ads on folded 8 1/2 by 11 white sheets of paper. I reported, interviewed, wrote, edited, photographed, and laid out each edition. I devised headlines, placed pull quotes, positioned pics, and wrote captions. I coordinated press runs and mail distribution with the printer. Yes, coworkers reviewed and edited my work, but for the most part, I was a one-man newspaper publisher.

I worked long hours on the tenth floor of the 9th and L Street building and worked long hours on the ground floor of the 13th and I Street building in downtown Sacramento. I learned my craft and produced fifty-six *California Publisher* editions during my five-year CNPA career.

One of my most noteworthy *California Publisher* accomplishments was single-handedly covering, from a newspapering perspective, a major regional disaster. On October 17, 1989, a 6.9 temblor, now known as the Loma Prieta earthquake, rocked seven San Francisco/Oakland Bay Area counties. In the days following the disaster, I called thirty-four of CNPA's member newspapers that were impacted by the earthquake. I interviewed publishers, newspaper executives or editors, compiled a report, and published that report in four pages of *California Publisher's* November 1989 edition. More than two years later, CNPA's Executive Director fired me because the association wanted to go in another editorial direction. That was the official reason. The catalyst that led to my termination was triggered when I asked for a pay raise.

After the spring 1992 Big Bear Landers earthquake/ Rodney King riots federally-declared disasters, the Governor's Office of Emergency Services (OES) hired me as a Reserve Information Officer (PIO) to work at OES' Disaster Field Office in Pasadena with other PIOs. I responded to media requests, communicated disaster relief information to the general public, analyzed news coverage, and edited the*Earthquake Safety Update*newsletter mailer.

In the fall of 1993/spring of 1994, I worked at the University of the Pacific (UOP) in Stockton's University Relations Office. My job was to promote the university. I was also Editor of UOP's alumni publication, *The Pacific Review*. I produced three editions of *The Pacific Review* during my stint at UOP.

The Department of Toxic Substances Control (DTSC) hired me to serve as a Public Participation Specialist (PPS). Even though I recorded textbooks for blind students at the California Department of Education's Clearinghouse Depository for Handicapped Students in the late seventies, worked as a Department of Housing Community Development student assistant in the mid-eighties, and served as a Governor's Office of Emergency Services Reserve Information Officer in the early nineties, I officially embarked on my state service career on May 5, 1994.

During my four-year tenure at DTSC, I helped form community Restoration Advisory Boards (RABs) and oversaw the implementation of public participation environmental cleanup programs at several closing and realigning military installations. I was DTSC's PPS at Alameda Naval Air Station (Alameda), Castle Air Force

Base (Atwater), China Lake Naval Air Weapons Station (Ridgecrest), and Mare Island Naval Shipyard (Vallejo).

I was hired as an Information Officer 1 at the Department of Motor Vehicles (DMV). While at DMV from 1998 to 2004, I was the editor of the *Spirit-Record*, the department's employee newspaper. I produced eighteen *Spirit-Record* issues—reporting DMV news, writing feature stories, taking photographs, laying out the paper with PageMaker desktop publishing software on an Apple computer, and working with the printer.

I pursued a lateral transfer at the California Community Colleges Chancellor's Office (CCCCO). I worked at CCCCO between 2004 and 2009.

One of my most noteworthy accomplishments at the Chancellor's Office was partnering with my California Department of Corrections and Rehabilitation (CDCR) and Palo Verde College (PVC) counterparts. In June 2007, we were involved with celebrating the largest number of inmates in the United States ever to earn higher education degrees at one time. The friends and families of inmates, plus college faculty, staff, corrections administrators, and community college guests attended this June 5, 2007, graduation.

Providing National Geographic Television's camera crew with information, arranging interviews, and coordinating video recording, my CDCR and PVC communications professional colleagues partnered with me in helping in the production of 2007"Lockdown" documentary. Because that episode was aired to millions of viewers nationwide, Community College Public Relations Organization awarded me the 2008 PRO Award for the media success story.

By the way, my CDCR counterpart was my elder sister, Terry Thornton. As far as I know, Terry and I were the first and only sibling PIOs in California state service. Terry was CDCR's Deputy Press Secretary until she retired on December 31, 2022.

Another noteworthy accomplishment at the Chancellor's Office was working with the office of then-Secretary of State Condoleezza Rice in the annual John W. Rice Diversity and Equity Awards. One of my duties as the CCCCO PIO was to help organize the presentation of the annual Rice Awards, established in 2001 to honor Dr. John W. Rice, Condoleezza Rice's late father. Dr. Rice served as a California Community Colleges Board of Governor. He died on December 24, 2000. So from 2005 to 2008, I'd routinely call Secretary Rice's office and ask Rice's secretary if she would attend the Rice Awards presentation. Because of Rice's national and international diplomatic demands, we knew she couldn't attend, but protocol necessitated that I/CCCCO make that perfunctory call anyway. Rice, through her secretary, would respectfully decline our invitation. My job then was to draft a statement about that year's Rice Awards' recipients, which I emailed to Rice's secretary, who then forwarded to Rice for Rice's approval. Rice's stepmother, Clara Bailey Rice, represented the late Dr. Rice and made the presentation.

More than a month after Rice resigned from her Secretary of State position, she was able to finally come to Sacramento in July 2009 and present the Rice Awards. It was an honor to finally meet Condoleezza Rice and take a picture with her.

I was promoted Information Officer 2 at the California Department of Public Health (CDPH). I started at CDPH on March 2, 2009. During my nearly fifteen-year tenure with this department—CDPH has responded to several health emergencies, such as swine flu/H1N1, hantavirus, Fukushima, Ebola, Zika virus, monkeypox (or MPX), and quite naturally, COVID-19.

Throughout the years, I have fielded hundreds of reporter inquiries about environmental health, family health, health equity, infectious diseases, and laboratory sciences, plus a lot more.

One of my most noteworthy media requests—involving laboratory sciences—was associated with Elizabeth Holmes. A federal jury convicted her for claiming to revolutionize blood testing. Holmes was convicted on four of eleven charges for defrauding investors while running Theranos Inc., which ended up as one of Silicon Valley's most notorious implosions, *The Wall Street Journal* (WSJ) reported on January 3, 2022.[27] That WSJ article further noted that the four-women and eight-men jury verdict put a punctuation mark on a scandal that surfaced with a series of WSJ articles in 2015 and 2016. Those articles called into question Theranos's proprietary blood-testing technology.

The downfall of Theranos and Holmes's conviction began when WSJ investigative reporter John Carreyrou queried CDPH's Office of Public Affairs (OPA) several times back in the summer of 2015. On July 16, 2015, the OPA Deputy Director back then asked me to "make sure this [Carreyrou's media request on laboratory company Theranos Inc.,] gets taken care of, please." In addition to querying OPA about Theranos, Carreyrou filed a California Public Records Act (PRA) request with CDPH.

---

[27] Michael Siconolfi, "Elizabeth Holmes to Report to Prison," The Wall Street Journal, updated May 26, 2023.

As a response to his PRA, CDPH's Laboratory Field Services (LFS) provided Carreyrou with 550 pages of responsive documents involving Theranos and Holmes. Carreyrou developed his WSJ reporting of Theranos and Holmes into a book titled *Bad Blood, Secrets and Lies in a Silicon Valley Startup*. The Theranos/Holmes story even became an international story when *60 Minutes Australia* did an exposé on Holmes in August 2021.

In an email I sent to OPA's Assistant Deputy Director, I stated, "Holmes' conviction was the result of Team CDPH (LFS, Office of Legal Services, OPA staff and Directorate); plus Agency (probably even the Governor's Office) throughout the years." I asked him to share all this with the Office of Comms team. But he did not do so, unless he shared with Deputy Director.

The other noteworthy incident that CDPH responded to was COVID-19. At the beginning of the pandemic, OPA staff worked at the Joint Information Center (JIC) at the Governor's Office of Emergency Services, located at the former Mather Air Force Base in Rancho Cordova. Most OPA staff members teleworked and provided web assistance from their respective domiciles.

In between routing media inquiries to the JIC, two other Information Officer 2s and I became a three-member quasi call center. The three of us answered a plethora of COVID-19 calls from the general public. At their end of their phone, we were the faceless voices who listened, responded to their questions, and in some cases, commiserated with and calmed them.

While working at my state job by day, I rewrote portions of the *Bible* in newspaper format (titled *The Testament Spectator*) at night, during the early morning hours, and on the weekend. The innovative idea of producing a *Bible* newspaper came to mind in the late eighties when I was the Publications Editor at the California Newspaper Publishers Association.

Thus, in October 1994, I produced my first four-page *Bible* newspaper edition and distributed *The Testament Spectator's* David and Goliath edition at Sacramento's 1994 Church Leadership and Sunday School (CLASS) Convention. CLASS was held at Capital Christian Center, located in east Sacramento. CLASS attendees well received The *Bible* newspaper concept. So throughout the years, I produced several more editions.

To date, I've rewritten about 10 percent of *The Holy Bible* in newspaper format. I've written *Testament Spectator* editions on Moses, the Hebrews' exodus from Egypt, and Red Sea crossing; Joshua and the Jericho conquest, Gideon and his victory against 150,000 Amalekites, Midianites, and their eastern allies; Samson and his supernatural muscular exploits; David and the entire book of 1 Samuel; the entire book of Jonah, a Hebrew prophet who resisted going to minister at Nineveh; and a 48-page/125-story amalgamated four-gospel edition on the life, times, and teachings of Jesus the Christ.

Anyone can download from my **www.Ronald FOwensJr.com** website *The Testament Spectator* in PDF at no cost. Those who do can email the PDF to a printer. Direct them to print the pages back-to-back in 11x17—or tabloid size paper—so *The Testament Spectator* can be read like reading a newspaper. *The Testament Spectator* would be great for home school, Sunday School or Vacation Bible School. Giving away *The Testament Spectator* is my gift for anyone who visits my website. Thank you for reading about me.

BIBLIOGRAPHY

1. Sarah Boseley and Melisa Davey, "Covid-19: Lancet retracts paper that halted hydroxychloroquine trials," The Guardian, June 4, 2020, <https://www.theguardian.com/world/2020/jun/04/covid-19-lancet-retracts-paper-that-halted-hydroxychloroquine-trials>.

2. Mandeep R Mehra, Frank Ruschitzka, Amit N Patel, "Retraction—Hydroxychloroquine or chloroquine with or without a macrolide for treatment of COVID-19: a multinational registry analysis," The Lancet, June 5, 2020, <https://www.thelancet.com/journals/lancet/article/PIIS0140-6736(20)31324-6/fulltext>.

3. Patrice Wendling, "Despite Retraction, Study Using Fraudulent Surgisphere Data Still Cited," Medscape Medical News, August 5, 2021, <https://www.medscape.com/viewarticle/956090?form=fpf>.

4. Ron Owens whistling the La Rèjouissance for Music | Royal Fireworks, by George Frideric Handel, last modified on April 12, 2013, <http://youtu.be/9dpLDhLUcwE>.

5. Ronald F. Owens Jr., <https://ronaldfowensjr.com>.

6. "It's simple. Does your chain link fence stop a mosquito," said Dr. Ramin Oskoui, CEO of Foxhall Cardiology, a Washington D.C.-based medical practice which specializes in internal medicine and cardiovascular disease, Facebook, July 15, 2020, <**https://www.facebook.com/604548277/posts/pfbidoNCdDqxsLVunUNHt9mTxRDDUycvVzKivVhJjn7tD8hpiabtNZdZC8YYoMR2gnvFXDl/?mibextid=cr9u03**>.

7. Dr. Pierre Kory, "Testimony of Pierre Kory, MD, Homeland Security Committee Meeting: Focus on Early Treatment of COVID-19," US Senate Homeland Security Committee, December 8, 2020, <**https://www.hsgac.senate.gov/imo/media/doc/Testimony-Kory-2020-12-08.pdf**>.

8. Front-Line COVID-19 Critical Care Alliance, (FLCCC) <**https://covid19criticalcare.com**>.

9. "White House Convening on Equity," The White House's YouTube channel, last modified April 14, 2022, <**https://youtu.be/_VhHno6REHM**>.

10. Ibid.

11. Vaccine Adverse Events Reporting System (VAERS), co-managed by the Centers for Disease Control and Prevention's (CDC), as of April 8, 2022, <**https://urldefense.com/v3/__https://openvaers.com/covid-data__;!!AvL6XA!iOQbqQTEgrhdTJopmLiXk3SFpgn-q7suqrAzZ83GX7lLTfIhh5N3DuOKaRRKzK_HBNH-dA$** >.

12. Ibid.

13. Ibid, as of October 3, 2022.

14. COVID VAERS Reports by STATE, States Summaries - OpenVAERS webpage. (<**https://openvaers.com/covid-data/states-summary**>.

15. Debora MacKenzie, "US smallpox vaccination plan grinds to a halt," New Scientist, August 22, 2003, <**https://www.newscientist.com/article/dn4074-us-smallpox-vaccination-plan-grinds-to-a-halt/**>.

16. Crutcher, Mark, director. "MAAFA 21: Black Genocide in 21st Century America," produced by Life Dynamics, 2009, <**http://www.maafa21.com/**>.

17. Sharp, Jennifer, director. "ANECDOTALS," Anecdotals, LLC, 2023, <**https://www.anecdotalsmovie.com**>.

18. Amy Kelly, "FOIA'd Emails Reveal Highest-Level Leaders at White House, HHS, CDC, NIAID, AAP All Knew COVID Vaccines Linked to Myocarditis, Yet Publicly Covered Up Findings," DailyClout, October 18, 2023, <**https://dailyclout.io/foiad-emails-reveal-highest-level-leaders-at-white-house-hhs-cdc-niaid-aap-all-knew-covid-vaccines-linked-to-myocarditis-yet-publicly-covered-up-findings/**>.

19. Booker T. Washington, Wikipedia, last edited on October 31, 2023, <**https://en.wikipedia.org/wiki/Booker_T._Washington**>.

20. Grand Jury The Court of Public Opinion, Berlin Corona Investigative Committee, <**https://grand-jury.net**>.

21. Ibid.

22. Ibid.

23. Rasmussen Reports, 2023, "Killer Jab? 24% Say Someone They Know Died From COVID-19 Vaccine," November 2, 2023, <**https://www.rasmussenreports.com/public_content/politics/public_surveys/killer_jab_24_say_someone_they_know_died_from_covid_19_vaccine**>.

24. SGT Report, "Pfizer & THE COVENANT WITH DEATH —DR. JAMES THORP," produced by SGT Report, November 8, 2023, <**https://rumble.com/v3uevrd-pfizer-and-the-covenant-with-death-dr.-james-thorp.html**>.

25. "ANECDOTALS," Anecdotals, LLC, 2023, <**https://www.anecdotalsmovie.com**>.

26. Did Mark Twain Say 'It's Easier to Fool People Than to Convince Them That They Have Been Fooled'?, Snopes, last modified on December 29, 2016, <**https://www.snopes.com/fact-check/did-mark-twain-say-its-easier-to-fool-people-than-to-convince-them-that-they-have-been-fooled/**>.

27. Michael Siconolfi, "Elizabeth Holmes to Report to Prison: A History of the WSJ Theranos Investigation, Holmes's downfall was triggered by these Wall Street Journal articles about the blood-testing company and its founder," The Wall Street Journal, updated May 26, 2023, <**https://www.wsj.com/articles/elizabeth-holmes-sentencing-a-history-of-the-wsj-theranos-investigation-11668741222**>.